TETRASOMA™ DIET FOR FOUR BODY TYPES

*Beneficial and Harmful Foods for Eastern
Yin Yang and Western Temperament Types*

By

David Lee, Ph.D., L.Ac.

TETRASOMA™ DIET FOR FOUR BODY TYPES
Copyright © 2015 by David Lee, Ph.D., L.Ac.

ISBN-13: 978-1511539289
ISBN-10: 1511539283

TABLE OF CONTENTS

ABOUT DAVID LEE

David Lee, Ph.D., is a licensed acupuncturist and an Asian herbal medicine practitioner. He received his doctorate of philosophy in Oriental medicine in 2006 from American Liberty University in Fullerton, California. In addition, he received his master's degree in Oriental Medicine in 1999 from Emperor's College of Traditional Oriental Medicine. He completed an externship at the Daniel Freeman Hospital in the city of Marina del Rey, California, and at the University of California Los Angeles Arthur Ashe Student Health and Wellness Center. He studied pre-medicine and received a bachelor of arts in psychology at University of California, Irvine. Dr. Lee has been practicing since 2000 and is currently based in Thousand Oaks, California.

Author of *Tetrasoma Diagnosis and Four Needle Technique, Tetrasoma Acupuncture Theory and Sasang Herbology, Tetrasoma Acupressure Therapy, Tetrasoma AcuMagnet Therapy,* and *Tetrasoma Case Review.*

ACKNOWLEDGEMENTS

My gratitude goes to the doctors who brought constitutional medicine to the global stage. And to my patient Elvira Wilson, whose loving heart and tenderness have spurred my realization that meaning, living, and health are intertwined.

DISCLAIMER

Patients are always encouraged to notify and work with their primary physician when making any health changes. This book is intended for food identification and elimination for the body type, and does not replace medical recommendations by your primary physician.

David Lee Acupuncture Clinic does not make any claims to diagnose, treat, or cure diseases that are not within the scope of acupuncture and Asian medicine. There is no guarantee that body type diet is for everyone, and not everyone will experience the same results.

Discontinue following the recommendations in this book if you experience dizziness, nausea, allergies, aggravation, or other unpleasant symptoms. Do not consume these foods if you have or have had life-threatening reactions with potential food allergens, such as nuts or shellfish.

FOREWORD

A holistic approach to health is becoming a more accepted approach to preventative care and treatment of chronic diseases. In conjunction, Eastern medicine is the fastest growing medical profession today.

For nearly 3,000 years, plant-based foods and herbs were some of the primary means of medicine for the treatment of acute, chronic, musculoskeletal, and internal diseases. Eastern medicine's theoretical framework and long medical history helped develop an efficient system for treating various ailments. Each patient is approached with the understanding that the individual's internal equilibrium and the body's illnesses need to be addressed simultaneously. By simply adjusting your body type through dietary changes, your body takes care of its own problems because its ability to maintain homeostasis is optimized.

Jema Lee, a Korean physician, presented Sasang Four Constitutional Medicine in 1894 as a quest to simultaneously increase longevity and health. He laid down a foundation of research that is recognized as an important step in furthering Asian medicine's efficacy. His accuracy is fueling its popularity today. He identified each body type through observation of the body shape, physiology, personality, food and herbal reaction, and disease process. Jema Lee's premise was that the treatment of diseases can be better customized for the individual when the inborn nature of the person is taken into consideration.

Tetrasoma^{TM} Body Type Diet is a partial fulfillment of Jema Lee's dream to bring medicine into every home. You can participate by understanding your body type's chemistry and adopting a diet that is best suited for you.

David Lee, Ph.D., L.Ac.
Doctor of Philosophy in Oriental Medicine
Licensed Acupuncturist

CHAPTER 1: BODY TYPE THEORY

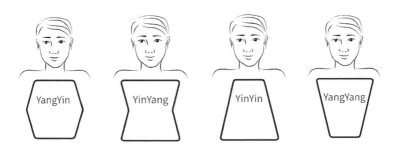

INTRODUCTION

A body type is a set of inborn physical, physiological, and psychological characteristics that distinguishes one group from another. The word 'body type,' or constitution, is a term used to group together and to distinguish a pool of individuals according to certain relevant and recurring similarities in their inherited qualities. There are many differences in the physical frame, physiology, and psychology that make us unique individuals. There are also common threads in the diverse gene pool that make some people respond in identical ways to certain stimuli. The body types are found in all ages, races, and sexes. There are four body types, each with their own health needs.

Determining what is appropriate and inappropriate for one's body type gives the individual the proper tools to actively participate in maintaining and improving health and preventing disease. Rather than relying on a problem-focused approach, a generalized body type diet focuses on the body's inherent ability to self-heal at multiple fronts. It awakens the body's own healing capacity to move toward a healthier state.

The benefits are holistic, without negative side effects. Good responses are obtained for all age groups, in acute to chronic conditions, and simple to complex diseases and conditions. The patient experiences not only relief from specific diseases, but the quality of the individual's life improves with less pain and inflammation, better sleep, increased energy, efficient body and clearer mind. The result is a greater sense of well-being.

The Yin Yang Body Type Diet focuses on the person rather than the disease. Even without a clear disease diagnosis, treating the person's body type can be enough to bring the body back into balance and to resolve the complaints. A person's body, especially at the beginning stage of a disease, has higher capacity to overcome illnesses. Tapping into this incredible innate ability is accomplished through empowering it to maintain its own natural homeostasis. Wrong food ingredients will inhibit the process of establishing the balance within.

Many diseases begin with years of subjective discomfort. They later manifest fully as outward symptoms and are positive on diagnostic examinations. When the body's imbalance is not severe, there is often no measurable difference; this imbalance may lie low for a long time. The only measureable indicator may be subjective discomfort or pain. Telltale signs and symptoms are often ignored until an actual problem arises or until the problem hampers the quality of daily living.

Body type diet does not replace the need to consult your physician nor medication when necessary. Presence of a disease indicates a seriousness of the ailment. It is used in conjunction with medical intervention to help the body restore its state of normal functioning. Even when diseases are well controlled with medications, the body is still in a dysfunctional state. Proper nutrition is necessary for the body to maintain health and well-being. Since many chronic diseases are originally created by unhealthy eating, they can be *reversed* by healthy eating.

BODY SHAPE CHARACTERISTICS

The majority of people have a body shape that is representative of their constitutions. Due to variation from person to person, however, the shapes represented here are not necessarily reflective of all individuals within a particular body type. The characteristics discussed below are overall tendencies and should not be used as definitive forms of identification.

Body Shape of a YangYin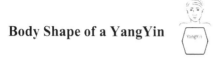

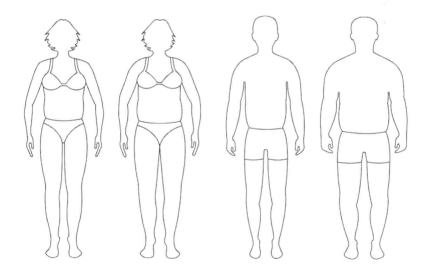

Figure 1

Other names: Apple Shape, Diamond Shape, Choleric, DiSC Dominance, Driving Style, Greater Yin and Lesser Yang combination, and GinLang.

7

- Muscles and Bones: Muscles are easily gained throughout the body with weight training. The lower half of the rib cage flares outward. Individuals within half of any given population tend to have bones that are larger than those of the other half.
- Weight Gain: Mesomorph to endomorph. The body is stout, easily gaining muscle and fat throughout. Weight gain is more prominent on the upper body in the shoulders, upper arms, back, chest, and abdomen. There is simultaneous protrusion of the upper and lower abdomen, as well as the sides of abdomen. The waist is curved outwards and is the widest part of the frame. There is more weight in the upper arms, upper buttocks, and upper legs compared to the lower part of the body.
- Proportion: Larger upper body, with wide upper back, larger upper arms, and ample bust. The majority of individuals with large chest and breasts are of this body type. Both the width of the shoulders at the acromio-clavicular joint and the upper hips are narrow compared to the mid-torso.
- Shoulders: Narrow and rounded.
- Hips: Narrower than the ribcage. Flatter buttocks.
- Feet: Wide.

Body Shape of a YangYang

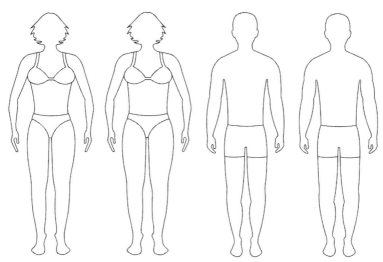

Figure 2

Other names: Triangle Shape, Down-Triangle Shape, Sanguine, DiSC Influence, Expressive Style, Greater Yang and Lesser Yang combination, and LangGang.

- Muscles and bones: It is not easy to gain muscle weight with weight training. Tends to have average or thinner bones.
- Weight gain: Ectomorph to mesomorph. Slim and thin. The majority of weight gain is in the trunk. Abdominal weight gain is noticeable mainly in front and less so on the sides. Both the upper and lower abdomen protrude evenly.
- Proportion: Larger upper body, with wide upper back and ample bust. Chest and upper back muscles are the first to develop with weight training.
- Shoulders: Broad, wide, straight, and squared.
- Ribcage: Narrow.
- Hips: Narrower than the ribcage. Flat hips and bottoms. Hips are slim and buttocks may have tendency towards flat side.
- Waist: Little curvature between the waist and hips.
- Feet: Narrow.

Body Shape of a YinYang

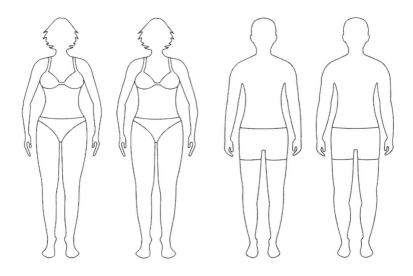

Figure 3

Other names: Hourglass, Bi-Triangle, Phlegmatic, DiSC Steadiness, Amiable Style, Lesser Yin and Greater Yang combination, and LinGang.

- Muscles and bones: Muscles do not bulk easily, even with exercise. Tends to have average or thinner bones.
- Weight gain: Ectomorph to mesomorph. Slim and thin. Extra weight is evenly distributed in the upper and lower body, although the initial gain is in the buttocks. The lower half of the abdomen, below the belly button, protrudes more than the upper.
- Proportion: The upper and lower body is evenly proportioned, separated by a curved-in waist.
- Shoulders: Straight, square, and wide.
- Ribcage: narrow.
- Hips: Wider than the ribcage.
- Feet: Narrow.

Body Shape of a YinYin

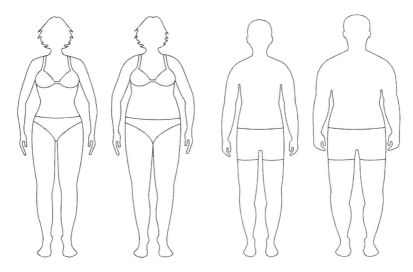

Figure 4

Other names: Pear Shape, Up-Triangle Shape, Melancholic, DiSC Conscientiousness, Analytical Style, Lesser Yin and Greater Yin combination, and LinGin.

- Muscles and bones: Stout muscles and strong bones. Muscles are evenly gained in both the upper and lower halves of the body, especially with weight training.
- Weight gain: Mesomorph to endomorph. There is more weight in the upper arms, upper and lower legs, abdomen, and buttocks. The first sign of weight gain is in the buttocks and lower half of body. Waist can be narrow or wide. Hips are larger than bust, and waist gradually slopes out to hips. Lower half of abdomen below belly button protrudes more than upper half.
- Proportion: The lower half of the body is larger and appears stronger.
- Shoulders: Rounded and narrower than hips.
- Ribcage: Lower half flares outward.
- Hips: Full. Wider than rib cage.
- Feet: Wide.

ORIGIN AND DEVELOPMENT OF ASIAN MEDICINE

The Asian medical system, based on a philosophy virtually unchanged since its inception, is coherent and well-reasoned Asian philosophy begins with the concept that all matter and movement in the universe have a common interaction. Just as electro-magnetism, gravity, strong nuclear force, and weak nuclear force are the fundamental laws in physics, yin-yang is the pure form of any matter, movement, direction, and thought, according to Asian medicine.

The unifying force of Tai-Chi (translated The Great Extreme) gives birth to two things: yin and yang. An old classical Chinese text[1] states that 'from one came two, from the two things came three, and from the three came the myriad of all things.' The Chinese feel that all complex matter can be reduced to simple, immutable law: yin and yang.

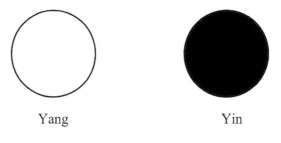

Yang   Yin

Figure 5

This dichotomy, polar opposite of yin, differentiates the two aspects. The above figures are symbols of yang as white and yin as black. Yin literally means the shadowy side of a hill and yang the sunny side of a hill. This binary point of view holds that there is always a counterpart, which is the direct opposite and at the same moment complementary. Where one exists, the other also resides. A male does not exist without a female, brightness does not exist without darkness, elation does not exist without sadness, upward does not exist without downward, and so on.

---

[1] The Way of Ethics, *Tao Te Ching*

The following lists some examples of yin and yang.

Table 1

YIN	YANG
shady side of hill	sunny side of hill
dark	bright
slow	fast
low	high
left	right
back	front
heavy	light
anger	joy
tail	head
rough	smooth
deficiency	excess

The items in the yin-yang categories are endless. There is nothing in the universe that does not have its fundamental component in either yin or yang. All physical objects, directions, movements, thoughts, and health are subject to the binary laws of yin and yang. Our mental processes require comparisons between opposing information to make sense of the world. Our physical movements require a fine balancing act between these opposing physical forces.

Since one complements the other, they are complete by being together as the following illustrates:

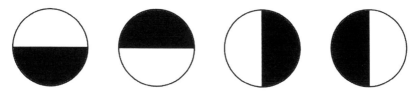

Balance: equal amount of yin and yang
Figure 6

The above symbols illustrate that the entire universe is made of half yin and half yang. 'From two came three' means that the third component of yin and yang is the middle line, or the point of differentiation. As can be seen in the same figure 6, there is a middle line that separates yin-black from yang-white. The circle represents wholeness, while differences exist within the confinement of the circle. The straight line within the circle means there is potential energy but there is no kinetic movement. Figure 7 illustrates the dynamic interaction between the two opposing forces:

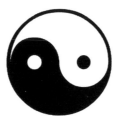

Active yin and yang
Figure 7

For example, if potential energy is night and day, then the transition from night to day and day to night is the active energy. The curved midline reflects the existence of movement, yin and yang playing tug of war. The two shapes inside the circle move in a clockwise direction, waxing, waning, and transforming into the other. The movement can also just as well be counter-clockwise, if the drawing is flipped.

There is nothing in the universe that does not have, in its essence, yin and yang. All physical objects, directions, movements, thoughts, and health are subject to the laws of yin and yang. Since the beginning of Eastern civilization, balance was an important aspect of health. The most authoritative ancient medical textbook[2], written over 2500 years ago, stresses the significance of being in balance and is still important today.

---

[2] Yellow Emperor's Classic of Medicine, *Huang Di Nei Jing*

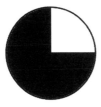 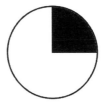

Too much yin   Too much yang
Not enough yang   Not enough yin

Figure 8

No one is born with perfect health because nobody has perfect balance of energies, even at birth. We are healthy when the energies within the body are within normal range. One can develop sickness when there is too much yang, not enough yin, too much yin, or not enough yang. The goal of treatment is to bring the amount of yin and yang to the equilibrium as shown in figure 7. If there is harmony of yin and yang, there is fullness of life. Grossly disproportionate yin and yang as illustrated in figure 8 is a state of disease. If severe, it can lead to a separation of yin (body) and yang (spirit). The result is inactivity and death, as shown in figure 5.

Ancient medical practitioners had limited knowledge of modern physiology, but they developed a medical system through clinical observations with application within their own framework. The result is the holistic medicine we enjoy today. Although the concept of yin and yang is surprisingly simple, there are infinite variations as reflected in the wide range of health and disease. A holistic approach is designed to treat multiple problems at once. Therefore, a theory of yin and yang can tackle this complexity and resolve multiple issues simultaneously.

Through meditative practices, ancient practitioners learned to discern proper from improper treatment. This practice is highly subjective and is therefore shunned by modern Western medicine. Asian medicine embraces both subjective experiences and objective observations. Trial and error was and still is part of medical evolution, but meditation and enlightenment has woven Asian medicine together as its own coherent system.

Meditation was a means of getting to know oneself and the world better. Individuals strove to divest themselves of factors that led to incorrect perception of the world. Those able to see the universe in its "true form," were considered enlightened. Their wisdom and proper advice were sought by the masses regarding government, economics, daily living, and health.

Those who were accomplished in meditation perceived the meridian energies flowing through channels within the body. The emotional, spiritual, and physical influence on the health of the human was visible to them. Stimulating the active points on the body with needles led to quicker recovery and over time these spots became known as acupuncture points. These first practitioners learned to identify and locate these acupuncture points, which have not changed for at least 3,000 years. These ancient sages also matched energetic properties of foods and herbs with the body to bring about right balance and to normalize the physiology.

FOUR BODY TYPES

The four body types are:
YangYin = Lesser Yang and Greater Yin combination
YangYang = Lesser Yang and Greater Yang combination
YinYang = Lesser Yin and Greater Yang combination
YinYin = Lesser Yin and Greater Yin combination

Each person is a combination of two of the four sub-body types:
1. Lesser Yang and Greater Yin (~25% of population)
2. Lesser Yang and Greater Yang (~25% of population)
3. Lesser Yin and Greater Yang (~25% of population)
4. Lesser Yin and Greater Yin (~25% of population)

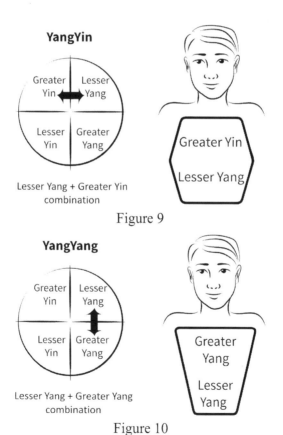

Figure 9

Figure 10

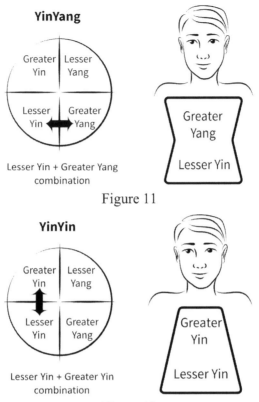

YinYang

Greater Yin | Lesser Yang

Lesser Yin | Greater Yang

Lesser Yin + Greater Yang combination

Greater Yang

Lesser Yin

Figure 11

YinYin

Greater Yin | Lesser Yang

Lesser Yin | Greater Yang

Lesser Yin + Greater Yin combination

Greater Yin

Lesser Yin

Figure 12

The incidence of Lesser Yin sub-body type is a majority in females (70~75% of all females) and the incidence of Lesser Yang sub-body type is a majority in males (70~75% of all males). These rates can vary from region to region but are a general trend.

A person with a sub-body type Lesser Yang may have either Greater Yang or Greater Yin as the other sub-body type. Similarly, a person with sub-body type Lesser Yin may have either Greater Yang or Greater Yin as the other sub-body type. Impossible combinations are:

- Lesser Yang + Lesser Yin
- Greater Yang + Greater Yin

Notice that Lesser Yang and Lesser Yin food lists are opposite to each other. Greater Yang and Greater Yin are also opposites. This is because these are opposite body types and they do not co-exist in an individual. A

Lesser Yang cannot be a Lesser Yin. And a person with Greater Yang cannot be a Greater Yin. So a combination of Lesser Yang with Lesser Yin is not possible. A Greater Yang combination with Greater Yin is also not possible.

The four body types Dr. Jema Lee proposed are Greater Yin, Greater Yang, Lesser Yin, and Lesser Yang, which are sub-body types under Tetrasoma theory. Each body type is defined based on the basic Asian philosophy of yin, yang, and the five elements: wood, fire, earth, metal, and water. Each of these words having many meanings is advantageous. Health can be dealt with in multiple ways using foods, which by nature have many facets.

Each person is composed of a fundamental and diverse nature of humanity but is distinct from others through body type differences. A Greater Yin body type's inherent state is an excessive (yang) wood and deficient (yin) metal energies. Its harmful foods aggravate the imbalance by further increasing the wood and further decreasing the metal while the beneficial foods do the opposite. Beneficial foods have a fine tuning effect toward the body's normal physiology, which constantly attempts to maintain homeostasis with biochemistry and anatomy. In the same respect, too much wood and too little metal will disrupt the normal functioning, creating low-grade problems and increasing susceptibility to diseases.

The three other sub-body types are also born with an imbalance of two of the five elements, carrying this asymmetry through one's lifetime. A Greater Yang body type has deficient (yin) wood and excessive (yang) metal energies, which are in opposite nature to the Greater Yins. For this reason, both Greater Yangs and Greater Yins cannot share their food lists. Harmful foods for one is beneficial for the other, and vice versa.

A Lesser Yang is born with an excessive (yang) earth and a deficient (yin) water energy. As with other body types, this discrepant state is set and will only be aggravated over time as we age. Proper foods and avoidance of harmful foods will enhance the quality, but will not reverse the process. The result of maintaining health and well-being through food management is still remarkable. A Lesser Yin has an opposite elemental states of deficient (yin) earth and excessive (yang) water, making the beneficial foods for Lesser Yang harmful and vice versa.

As the constitutional system has become refined since the 19th century, it is increasingly apparent that everyone has a paired combination of the above four as sub-body types, still ending up as four body types.

The following chart identifies the five elemental states of each body type. The body type diet automatically adjusts the discrepancy of the five elements, leading to a more balanced body.

Table 2

4 Body Types	Wood	Fire	Earth	Metal	Water
YangYin	high	high	high	low	Low
YangYang	low	low	high	high	Low
YinYang	low	low	low	high	high
YinYin	high	low	low	low	high

Excessive (high) and deficient (low) states of the five elements above indicate a basic innate state of imbalance within each body type. It recognizes each body type group's differing needs to maintain good health. No person is in a complete balanced state. Neither is better than the other since there are both advantages and disadvantages.

Chapter 3 will have questionnaires and descriptions of the four sub-body types to help assess which two sub-body types you belong to.

CHAPTER 2: FOODS FOR THE BODY TYPE

The foods that we eat everyday have tremendous impact on our health. Food should not only provide nutrition and calories for energy, but also serve as medicine that affects the way our body functions. Food is an indispensable part of healing and can be used in a proactive way to keep people responsible for their own health.

Before bio-molecular medicine became dominant, herbs were used to treat diseases because they strongly influence the body's physiology. Food and herbs have the same source, the former being more nutritious and the latter being more medicinal. Because we consume foods every day, over time their effects can accumulate in our bodies for health or for harm.

Many diseases can be avoided and treated simply by changing our diets. Many people turn from destructive eating habits after seeing loved ones suffer from debilitating or terminal diseases. Heart disease, liver disease, kidney disease, diabetes, recurrent infection, and digestive problems are still rampant. Obesity causes and aggravates many diseases. They can be prevented by eating foods that promote optimal health benefits to the body.

Improved digestive function, moods, hormonal balance, energy, and sense of well-being are all subjective experiences that suggest the body's healthier state.

> Many diseases can be avoided and treated simply by avoiding harmful foods for the body type.

Peanuts, tree nuts, dairy, gluten, soybeans, eggs, chicken, garlic, onion, corn, and shellfish are not only common foods, but are also common in being beneficial or harmful due to their ubiquity. The harm or the benefit depends on the individual's body type, not the food itself. Food allergies and intolerance are genetically expressed. A person can be harmed or benefited by the same foods throughout their lifetime. As we age, it is increasingly imperative to avoid foods that cause stress to our bodies.

FOOD ALLERGY-INTOLERANCE

There are three characteristics of food that one should be aware of and practice regularly. They are allergy-intolerance, variety-moderation, and toxicity-cleanliness. This book discusses the allergy-intolerance for each body type. Allergy-intolerant foods elicit an immune system response and create stress for the body's normal physiology due to a mismatch with the body

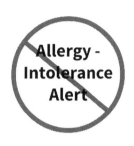

type. Rather than promoting health, they wreak havoc, especially in a weakened state. Because their harmful effects are subtle and minute, they are wrongly deemed safe. For this reason, they are still ubiquitous and commonly consumed. The hypersensitivity can be reduced by the body getting used to them, but continual consumption will inhibit its normal functioning. They make the body more difficult to come back from injuries and worsen age-related illnesses. Since the negative response is an expression from your genetic make-up, they should either be avoided or minimized.

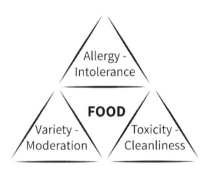

Figure 13

Variety-moderation relates to the diversity of nutrients that the body requires for maintaining normal function and storing them in reserve for its future use, thereby consistently promoting a healthier body. Body type diet does not restrict your diet, but is an adjustment through providing additional ingredients you would not consume otherwise. It provides diversity of foods for the body's requirement and for your enjoyment. A habit of consuming low variety will result in nutritional deficiency increasing susceptibility for diseases and hastening the aging process, especially if the foods are starchy and fatty.

Toxicity-cleanliness refers to foods that are laced with unnatural chemicals or some GMOs (Genetically Modified Organisms) forcibly causing harmful effects. Some toxic chemicals are artificial flavoring, artificial coloring, pesticides, and preservatives. Many industrial chemical by-products are not bio-degradable and will be inadvertently present in the foods. A solution to efficiently produce crops for the growing world population is leading to increased development of GMOs, which may have unintended consequences to the environment and to our health.

To test which foods are harmful, start by identifying the foods you suspect to be the culprits. Completely avoid one food item for an entire week and then introduce it in significant amount with every meal for two to three days. Observe and note the body's response in this 48-72 hour period. Repeat with other foods. It may require a longer period of consumption for your physiology to exhibit negative symptoms. Repeat several times to observe and confirm through consistent negative responses. *Caution: do not consume any food if you are known to be hyper-allergic or intolerant. You may go into anaphylactic shock, which is a life-threatening reaction.*

Avoiding or minimizing harmful foods is more important than eating the right foods because the health-promoting foods will not cancel out the negative impact of harmful foods. So it is best not to introduce the harmful ingredients in the first place.

FOOD ITEMS FOR THE BODY TYPE

Each body type recognizes a unique set of beneficial and harmful foods. Your body is a combination of two out of four different body types and will receive benefit or harm when you eat any of the foods from these categories. You should fill out the questionnaire to determine which two body types you are. Knowing what to eat for your body type is a helpful guide to consuming the right foods, while avoiding harmful foods.

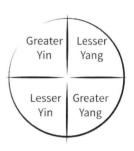

2 sub-body types
make 1 body type

The following lists are common foods specific to the four body types and are known to have a strong impact on health. Many other common food items are not mentioned in this book because they can be consumed by all four body types. In these cases, the negative/positive effects of such foods are so mild that they are close to being neutral and the long term effects are negligible. Some food items are not mentioned because they are not commonly consumed, or the influence on the body types are not known. The degree of negative and positive impact may vary, depending on the food item and the individual.

When deciding to make changes to your diet, a significant change with at least 70% reduction of the harmful foods from your current diet and adding the beneficial foods to your daily meal is, in most cases, practical and sufficient. A complete elimination of harmful foods is in most cases impractical because of ubiquitous presence in many processed foods. And these common foods have been deemed generally safe through generations. If those ingredients do not cause a severe or a life-threatening reaction, then the small amount is not enough to trigger a meaningful reaction even when taken over a period of time. Once you see the negative reaction, it is a cue to cut down the harmful foods from your diet.

Eating only the beneficial foods listed below without eating a variety of foods is not recommended. The following list is not comprehensive, but contains foods that are known to strongly influence the body's physiology over time, albeit subtle. To have diversity of nutrients, the beneficial foods should be incorporated along with many other nutritious foods.

Often, the subtle negative impact of harmful foods can be more dangerous to health than those that cause immediate reactions. When the effect of harmful foods is immediately noticeable or measurable, it provides a clear reason to either reduce or eliminate them. Because the constant presence of mildly harmful foods causes subtle changes, the identification harmful foods as the real cause of the disease is elusive. An eventual disruption of the body's normal physiology with dysfunction of organs and an inability to recover is only a matter of time.

Not all food ingredients on the lists below have equal impact on the body. The degree of influence is dependent on the ingredient and the receptivity of the body. The negative impact of some ingredients is quick and strong. Nuts, dairy, fish, shellfish and soy are known to be highly allergic-intolerant to some. Others are more subtle and take longer time to cause havoc. Such are seemingly innocuous lettuce and cabbage, which can cause fatigue without presence of other intolerant symptoms for Greater Yins if consumed in large amounts for a long period. For these individuals, their salads should consist of other vegetables.

The symptoms from the same food can vary individually. For example, one Greater Yang sub-body type will have strong intolerant reaction to dairy with mild reaction to nuts. Another individual of the same sub-body type will have anaphylactic response to nuts but will not notice ill-effect from dairy.

Harmful foods do not have to be avoided altogether. It is difficult to do so at times when beneficial foods are unavailable or there is sporadic craving for the harmful foods. A small amount, which is a 70-80% reduction of your current intake, can be supportive toward health and well-being by providing variety of nutrients. But a moderate to large amount consumed on a regular basis will eventually make the body unable to process them out efficiently and to function properly at its optimal level. When you significantly reduce harmful foods from your diet, you naturally choose the beneficial and neutral foods.

Most ingredients not listed in this book are likely neutral or mild in their effect on the body type. Since they are beneficial for everyone, they can be consumed regularly without causing any long term problem.

If you suspect or know some foods cause side effects or life-threatening reactions, do not consume them.

Lesser Yang Sub-Body Type Foods

Harmful Foods
Grain - brown rice, corn (whole, syrup, starch), Meat - chicken Fruit - apple, tangerine, orange, grapefruit, lime, lemon Spice* - warming spices such as ginger, garlic, chili, fennel, black pepper, turmeric, cinnamon, cayenne Supplement – honey, ginseng

Beneficial Foods
Bean - azuki bean, mung bean, mung bean sprout, pea, snap pea, snow pea Fish - most fresh and salt water fish Fruit – cooling fruits such as strawberry, raspberry, blackberry, watermelon, honey dew, cantaloupe, cactus fruit, banana Gluten** - gluten containing grains such as wheat, rye, barley, oat Meat - small to moderate amounts of pork, turkey, duck), egg white Spice – cooling spices such as in mint family Supplement – aloe Vegetable - celery, cucumber, eggplant, cactus leaf

* Spices should not be consumed for therapeutic benefit but small amount for food flavoring is not harmful. Most spices, which are warming, should be minimized. However, cooling spices in the mint family, such as mint, basil, rosemary, sage, oregano, and can be consumed. Overconsumption of mint may relax the esophageal sphincter, causing acid reflux.

** Gluten is not harmful. Gluten is contained in some grains, which are starchy with carbohydrates, and should be consumed in moderate or lower amount.

All body types do well with chlorella, chia seed, hemp seed, and spirulina, which are excellent sources of protein with complete amino acids. Most people can reduce harmful foods by 70% without harmful effect. This means one can keep variety of ingredients in meals.

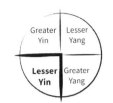

Greater Yin | Lesser Yang
Lesser Yin | Greater Yang

Lesser Yin Sub-Body Type Foods

Harmful Foods

Bean - azuki, mung
Fruits - strawberry, raspberry, blackberry, watermelon, honey dew cantaloupe, banana
Grain - gluten containing grains such as wheat, rye, barley, oat
Meat - pork, egg white, duck
Spice – cooling spices such as mint, basil, oregano, rosemary, sage
Supplement - succulents such as aloe vera, cactus, cactus fruit
Vegetable – celery stalk, celery root, cucumber, eggplant

Beneficial Foods

Fruit - apple, tangerine, orange, lemon, grapefruit
Grain – gluten free grains in moderation amaranth, corn, millet, montina, quinoa, rice, sorghum, teff, etc.
Meat - small to moderate amount of chicken, lamb, goat
Spice – warming spices such as ginger, garlic, curry, thyme, dill, fennel, black pepper, mustard, turmeric, cayenne
Supplement – apple cider vinegar, ginseng, royal jelly, honey

Pointer #1: Some Lesser Yins have stomach pains with shellfish. Lesser Yins are not allergic to corn, but it is starchy. Soy is a legume, which indicates that some Greater Yangs may have an allergic reaction.

All body types do well with chlorella, chia seed, hemp seed, and spirulina, which are excellent sources of protein with complete amino acids. Most people can reduce harmful foods by 70% without harmful effect. This means one can keep variety of ingredients in meals.

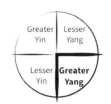

Greater Yang Sub-Body Type Foods

Harmful foods
Bean – all legumes in moderate to high amount Dairy - milk, cheese, yogurt, whey Meat - large amounts of egg yolk, beef, chicken, lamb, sheep, pork, venison such as deer, moose, elk, reindeer, buffalo, caribou, and antelope Nut and Seed - walnut, almond, cashew, pistachio, macadamia, sunflower seed, chestnut, pumpkin seed, brazil nut Oily and Fried Foods – moderate to high amount Spice - onion Supplement - coffee Vegetable – artichoke, leek Vegetable – root vegetables such as radish, turnip, parsnip, sweet potato, yam

Beneficial foods
Fish – all fish (fresh and salt water), all shellfish such as shrimp, clam, crab, oyster, sea urchin Fruits - cherry, grape, kiwi Grain – buckwheat Vegetable – all surficial (above ground) vegetables. All lettuce such as iceberg and romaine, all cabbage family such as broccoli, brussels sprouts, cabbage, cauliflower, some root vegetables such as beet, carrot

All body types do well with chlorella, chia seed, hemp seed, and spirulina, which are excellent sources of protein with complete amino acids. Most people can reduce harmful foods by 70% without harmful effect. This means one can keep variety of ingredients in meals.

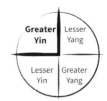

Greater Yin Sub-Body Type Foods

Harmful foods
Fish - all shellfish such as shrimp, clam, crab, oyster, sea urchin Fruit - persimmon Grain - highly starchy* foods such as corn, grains, white potato Vegetable - all lettuces such as romaine, iceberg, red leaf. all cabbage family such as broccoli, brussels sprouts, cabbage, cauliflower, collards, kale, kohlrabi

Beneficial foods
Bean – most beans such as coffee**, cacao, peanut, chickpea, lentil, kidney, lima, fava, garbanzo, black, pinto Meats – beef, venison such as deer, moose, elk, reindeer, buffalo, caribou, and antelope Dairy*** - milk, cheese, yogurt Fruit - blueberry, pear, plum Nuts and Seed – all nuts and seeds such as peanut, walnut, almond, brazil, cashew, pistachio, macadamia, chestnut, sunflower seed, chia seed, flax seed, pine nut Spice – leek, onion Vegetable - many surficial vegetables such as spinach, leek, artichoke, asparagus, pumpkin, squash, zucchini. most root vegetables such as radish, carrot, parsnip, rutabaga, turnip, yam, sweet potato, maca, taro, lotus root, leek, jicama, burdock root. seaweed****

* Greater Yins do not do well with high carbohydrate diet. Highly starchy foods such as corn, wheat, rye, barley, and white potato have to be significantly reduced although they are not allergic or intolerant to them. They should be limited to small amount, while carbohydrates from fruits and vegetables should be their main source.

** Coffee and other caffeinated teas are beneficial for YangYin (Lesser Yang and Greater Yin combination) and can have up to two or three servings a day. But both YinYin (Lesser Yin and Greater Yin combination) and YinYang (Lesser Yin and Greater Yang combination) are hypersensitive to caffeine with inability to sleep soundly. YangYangs (Lesser Yang and Greater Yang combination) are not as sensitive as Lesser Yins but will cause dehydration leading to multiple problems. Limiting caffeine to one serving only in the morning is suggested.

*** Dairy is beneficial for Greater Yins but a regular consumption in moderate to large amount will inhibit normal physiology. Many YinYins (Lesser Yin and Greater Yin combination) do not do well with dairy because Lesser Yin sub-body type aspect tends to be intolerant to dairy.

**** Seaweed is most beneficial for a YangYin (Lesser Yang and Greater Yin combination). Some Lesser Yins are intolerant to it.

All body types do well with chlorella, chia seed, hemp seed, and spirulina, which are excellent sources of protein with complete amino acids. Most people can reduce harmful foods by 70% without harmful effect. This means one can keep variety of ingredients in meals.

SIDE EFFECTS OF HARMFUL FOODS

Note the foods that adversely affect you. The negative side effects of such foods can include:

☐ bloating

☐ continuous coughing

☐ diarrhea

☐ eczema/skin reaction

☐ headache

☐ heaviness

☐ indigestion

☐ inflammation or raw sensation in the lips or tongue

☐ nasal discharge

☐ nausea

☐ short of breath

☐ sleepiness

☐ sneezing

☐ swelling

☐ tiredness

☐ yawning

The unpleasant effects of some harmful foods are immediately noticeable even with small amounts. Others are manifested over time or through the process of elimination. It may be more difficult to notice the positive effects of beneficial foods because it is easier to recognize discomfort and displeasure. If you are sure that one or two of the food ingredients in the lists are harmful to you, then the rest of the foods in the box are also harmful in varying degrees. If you have identified several ingredients in each of two harmful food lists of the four sub-body type categories, then you may be that body type combination.

You may have yet to notice the negative impacts of other foods in the same harmful category. For example, a person who has a known peanut allergy is also allergic to other nuts and is intolerant to dairy products, although there may be no perceivable symptoms from eating these. If they are only suspects, then other identified foods in the same list help to confirm them as harmful as well.

Non-organic and GMO foods can aggravate the effects of already harmful ingredients or mask the effect of beneficial foods. The modern alteration of foods has made the foods drastically different, in many cases harmful. They are genetically altered, creating a potential for many unknown side effects. Many are void of nutrients. Pesticides used to kill unwanted insects are in turn causing harm to our bodies. Be mindful of consuming organic and non-GMO foods while testing the ingredients on yourself.

The positive side effects of consuming beneficial foods are multi-fold. Any single food item is complex. Even one nutrient has many effects. The goal is to consume foods that affect the body in many positive ways at once. This holistic approach has been observed since ancient times and deserves respect. The foods having the quality as warming, cooling, drying, dampening, draining, and dispersing is a way to convey the observation of multiple effects of a single food item under a common thread. Whereas scientific medicine searches understanding through a specific pathway while attempting to minimize other effects, a holistic approach looks at the whole picture and provides application to fit the picture. As many effects as possible are desired as long as they are positive.

The positive side effects of foods are opposite to the negative side effects. Positive effects of beneficial foods are:

> Gluten intolerance is often associated with irritable bowel syndrome and is solely found in Lesser Yin sub-body types. The best solution is to avoid it. Gluten is a cereal protein mainly found in wheat, rye, barley and to a lesser degree in oats. Most commonly, it is an autoimmune system reaction that leads to mal-absorption in the intestines and causes irregular bowel movement. Other reactions are fatigue, foggy memory, slurred speech, and arthritic pains. Gluten intolerance is more prevalent in females than in males.

☐ feeling healthier and stronger
☐ regulated bowel
☐ sleep more soundly
☐ energy increased
☐ lightness in mind and body
☐ increased stamina
☐ lessened disease symptoms
☐ lessened low grade symptoms

☐ upright spine, less slouching
☐ easier to smile and laugh
☐ increased enjoyment
☐ more focused
☐ improved clarity
☐ improved memory
☐ less infections
☐ less experience of stress

FOODS AND HEALTH

Foods have a strong influence on our health. Apart from providing nutrition and energy, the health influence of food can be subtle and strong. Beneficial foods can be used to improve our health—but foods can be detrimental to health if the ones consumed are wrong for the body type. Benefit *or* harm occurs depending on *who* is consuming it.

Harmful foods have a very subtle impact on most people so there is difficulty recognizing them as being negative. Even if there are negative symptoms, these are seen as inconveniences rather than precursors to major diseases. The unpleasant experience is only the tip of the iceberg; there may be a series of physiological events that are difficult to identify but nonetheless present.

Personal beliefs or negative experiences unrelated to negative physiological responses are not a realistic gauge to determine which foods are right for you. Social, cultural, and psychological factors influence the visual, olfactory, taste and texture preferences. The body, however, acts independently from these influences, according to its biological needs.

Some healthy comfort foods are often mistakenly seen as beneficial. Chicken soup and traditional family dishes have a nostalgic appeal and produce psychological satisfaction. Just because they are low in calories, not greasy, and not fattening does not mean they equate to being healthy. They are marginally safe enough to be widely consumed around the world across many groups for energy and nutrition. But if they happen to be inappropriate for your body type, then there will be a temporary or long-term negative consequence.

Constant, long-term ingestion of even the most commonly consumed foods will harm the body over time if they are not right for the body type. Consumption on a daily or near daily basis will compromise the body quicker. The effects are so subtle and mild that the impact is gradual to the point where the body cannot process out the harmful foods anymore. They build up over time and wreak havoc, leading toward sickness and/or aggravating diseases. For this reason, unrecognized harmful foods can do great harm.

Infants and children are highly sensitive to foods. When the body does not like certain foods, there is vomiting, diarrhea, eczema, asthma, and nasal discharge. As they grow older, this defense mechanism becomes dull and we misperceive the lessening of negative reaction as growing out of them. But the perceived reactions are only the tip of the iceberg, and underneath there is a harmful impact on the physiology that manifests itself as diseases later in adults. Childhood diseases and seemingly harmless discomforts may turn into chronic diseases if ignored.

Nuts, seeds in the nut category, dairy, corn, corn syrup, corn starch, onion, and chicken are some top harmful foods for the YangYangs (Lesser Yang and Greater Yang combination). Just by eating chicken regularly, this body type can aggravate the intensity and frequency of hot flashes related to menopause. It can also cause chronic fatigue and cause one to become prone to emotional outbursts. For this reason, one cannot blame ailments on uncontrollable factors. Food is a significant contributor to our health. Choosing the right type of foods is within our control.

Because the harmful foods are commonly and regularly consumed, they are the cause of chronic problems. They are often recurrent infections,

A low carbohydrate diet is especially beneficial for the Greater Yin body types in combination with Lesser Yang or Lesser Yin. Consumption of sugar, grains, corn, and white potato should be sporadic. In addition to increased physical stamina and mental clarity, many find that just lowering simple carbohydrates reduces symptoms of chronic diseases such as yeast infections, migraines, asthma, high blood glucose and sinus congestion.

seasonal or all-year-round allergies, stomach pains, irritable bowel symptoms, fatigue, lack of motivation, difficult focusing, low grade scores, and missing school often. Stimulants and quick picker-uppers temporarily mask the underlying issues. The only means of improvement is to minimize or to avoid these foods.

Most of the time, strong adverse effects such as allergic reactions or anaphylaxis do not occur. Anaphylaxis is characterized by breathing obstruction, drop in blood pressure, internal bleeding, and shock. Less intense manifestations are the general subjective experience of pain, along with compromised sleep, digestion, circulation, stamina, clarity of thought, and general sense of well-being, and enjoyment of daily activities.

Even with proper medical treatments, avoidance of harmful foods is often essential for a successful recovery. So if you have unexplained subjective symptoms of general malaise, bloating, fatigue, and headache, then begin eliminating harmful foods from your diet. Minimizing or eliminating medical intervention is possible through good diet that promotes health and well-being.

Although age and propensity are factors in maintaining good health, most people do not have optimal health because the bodies break down

An eight year old child came home from school at least 3 times a month with stomach cramps and severe allergic rhinitis. These symptoms were a daily occurrence since infancy. Skin and blood allergy tests did not reveal any possible food culprit. As a YangYang body type (Lesser Yang + Greater Yang combination), the harmful foods were requested to be significantly reduced or eliminated. At the end of three weeks, 90% of symptoms were gone. By this time, most of the harmful food items were not present in the body. The improved state maintained as long as the diet for the body type was observed.

prematurely. Many chronic diseases occur in later years but are not unavoidable if one sticks to the body type diet. Foods have a large role in maintaining optimal health for one's age. Just by adjusting to one's own needs, there can be significant improvement and greater stability. The ability to buffer from daily stressors is then maximized.

Meals come in innumerable combinations, amounts, and varieties so there is almost no opportunity to test one food at a time. If we could eat one food item at a time as a meal, then the task of distinguishing harmful from beneficial would be much simpler. A practical method is to repeat the same ingredient at each normal meal for several days to identify the harmful food. Most processed foods found in groceries or restaurants are not prepared for any body type. These combinations make us constantly exposed to inappropriate ingredients. Healthy combinations of food for each body type is not feasible outside of home, especially for the

YangYang body type (Lesser Yang and Greater Yang combination). They may have to resort to preparing their own meals.

Asian medicine is holistic and the foods are studied in whole forms as they affect the body in multiple ways. It is a one-food-fits-whole type of approach. Scientific findings are helping to confirm the relationship between body types and the harmful foods. Specific ingredients found in foods such as gluten, lactose, casein, and corn protein contribute to understanding the mechanism of how molecular components act against normal body physiology.

The harmful foods do not have to be avoided altogether. We have eaten most of the foods listed above at one time or another, with minimal negative impacts. Consuming manageable amounts of harmful food is acceptable as long as the body can render them harmless. The prevalence of hidden harmful foods makes it difficult to eliminate them from our diet. Making significant changes is therefore sufficient and practical.

FOOD AMOUNT VS. FOOD TYPE

More does not mean better. Having a buffet style meal everyday leads to indigestion and overworking the body. Overeating beneficial foods will also do the same. Avoiding harmful foods may reduce the food choices, but many varieties are still available. A lack of nutrients should be of no concern. Antioxidants, vitamins, fiber, trace minerals, and other nutrients are all necessary for the proper functioning of human body. Our bodies know how to utilize the nutrients in foods optimally when they are comfortable with the whole food that is being ingested. So the food items are just as important as the nutrients contained within. Foods that are good for the body type enhance the vital role in health, which includes memory, longevity, mood, circulation, maintenance, homeostasis, recuperation, and immune responsiveness.

DETOXIFICATION AND WEIGHT CONTROL

Excessive eating and accumulation of harmful substances necessitate routine detoxification. The overload burdens the body's normal functioning and defense mechanisms. Many of us need to release the excess from flesh, circulatory system, and organs. Those with intractable diseases such as diabetes, fibromyalgia, and cancer notice improvement, while others with lesser discomforts can use a detoxification diet for prevention. On average, a detoxification diet every three months for a period of one week should be sufficient if you are already on a healthy body type diet.

The detoxification diet consists of fruits and vegetables. The kinds are different for each of the four body types. Combining two of the four food categories listed below works best because every person is composed of two body types. The symptoms of improvement include more energy, curved appetite, and improvement of diseases.

Lesser Yang Sub-Body Type
Blackberry, watermelon, honey dew, cantaloupe, cucumber, celery, eggplant, mung bean, mung bean sprouts, and strawberries.

Lesser Yin Sub-Body Type
Soy bean, maple syrup, apple, orange, pomegranate, and lemon. Hot spices such as cayenne pepper, garlic, black pepper, chili pepper, turmeric, cinnamon, and ginger.

(Some Lesser Yins have sensitive stomach with spices manifesting as abdominal cramping or acid reflux. If so, the spices should be introduced in small amounts over time to desensitize the body. The abdominal discomfort will go away and the health benefits of these ingredients will take place.)

Greater Yang Sub-Body Type
Broccoli, brussels sprouts, cabbage, cauliflower, iceberg lettuce, white grapes, cherry, kiwi, kale, romaine lettuce, and leafy greens.

Greater Yin Sub-Body Type
Pears, plums, onion, nuts, legume, leeks, pumpkin and squash. Root vegetables such as burdock, carrot, turnip, parsnip, radish, maca, taro, jicama, rutabaga, platycodon, sweet potato, lotus root, and yam.

Avoid animal meat, greasy foods, and grains while on this diet. The amount and calories should equate to regular meals. They can be prepared raw or cooked in a combination that is tasteful to you. But at least half the ingredients should be raw to prevent destruction of some essential nutrients cooked in high heat. Do not continue if you experience dizziness, severe weakness, or allergic symptoms. If these food selections are too limited for you, then the regular avoidance of harmful foods is still sufficient to gently detoxify. This will eliminate the need for routine detoxifying diet. In addition, consuming low animal protein and sticking to mainly fruits and vegetables will add quality years to your health and life.

Plant source proteins such as chia seed, quinoa, hemp seed, and chlorella are excellent and are neutral for all body types. Spirulina, a cyanobacteria, is also an optimal source of protein.

CHAPTER 3: BODY TYPE DIAGNOSIS

IMPORTANCE OF BODY TYPING

Each body type progresses toward and responds to identical diseases differently. For this reason, the one-size-fits-all approach cannot be applied in medicine. Side effects attest to the fact that human physiology is not identical across the population. While many will improve, others will only slightly improve, and still others will experience no improvement along with severe side effects. Therefore, there is a need to provide individualized treatments while treating the diseases themselves. Medicine evolves to better recognize and deal with the human variation. It strives to understand the disease etiologies, to avoid unnecessary applications, and to apply correct treatments.

Constitutional medicine is the missing link that helps us understand the response variations to diseases and treatments. It takes inborn variation as the chief consideration before deciding on the treatment of the disease. Identifying the normal states and the congenital imbalances of the individual provides customized treatments. As a result, the desired outcome is easier to achieve and is more reliable.

BODY TYPING IN FOUR CONSTITUTIONAL MEDICINE

Each of the four body types in the Four Constitutional Medicine has distinctive traits from another—physiologically, pathologically, and psychologically. These traits manifest in the outer physical appearance, body functions and personalities.

The following conditions listed are designed for an easy determination of your body type. You may find items on one list that more strongly reflect you than another. If so, they may describe your body type. First, match yourself against the Greater Yang and Greater Yin sub-body types. After identifying the one that is overall more similar to you, go onto the next two lists, which are Lesser Yang and Lesser Yin sub-body types. The two lists with the highest running total may be your body type.

Any sub-body type traits can occur in all the body types, but it is more likely to appear in its pertaining body type. Everyone can develop the symptoms on the list at one time or another. This is because we all have varying propensities to manifest these symptoms. Instead of linking the traits to one or two specific incidences, observe yourself across many situations by placing yourself in the third person and measuring yourself against the general population. Then decide where your tendency lies. If unsure, do not mark the boxes.

Influences of cultural, social, and personal background make some elements of the list difficult to understand, vague, or misleading. However,

A female YangYang body type (Lesser Yang + Greater Yang combination) patient had severe lack of sleep in the past 3 weeks due to intense hot flashes. They occurred several times an hour during day and night. She was health conscious about organic foods and eating well-balanced diet but wondered why her hormones were raging. On removal of chicken, however, her hot flashes had diminished significantly within a few days and her quality sleep had returned.

the number of questions is expansive enough for you to determine your body type. The detailed explanation of the questionnaire in the next section is helpful in clarifying its meaning. Comprehensive examination by an experienced Four Constitutional Medicine practitioner can help confirm your body type diagnosis.

Greater Yang and Greater Yin sub-body types are opposite to each other in physiology and in mental processes. Lesser Yang and Lesser Yin sub-body types also have opposite characteristics. Although we are all human, the way each individual's body works is different. Try to understand your body type in relation to your healthy state, not when you were sick or fighting an illness.

There are no preferable or advantageous body types. Each has its own strengths and weaknesses. Like two sides of a coin, each body type has positive traits, as well as undesirable characteristics. Human bodies are complex and dynamic. What can be disadvantageous in one situation can be highly desirable in another.

Some descriptions of body type characteristics are stereotypical to convey a clearer picture. Objectively evaluate yourself against the body type characteristics and see where your tendencies lie.

SELF-DIAGNOSIS

After you have marked the boxes that apply to you in the following sections, tally up the numbers. The two boxes with the highest total count indicate your body type combination. A difference between the totals of two sub-body types (Lesser Yang vs. Lesser Yin, and Greater Yang vs. Greater Yin) by four or less may not provide an accurate diagnosis.

	total count		total count
Lesser Yang (a)	⬜	Greater Yang (c)	⬜
Lesser Yin (b)	⬜	Greater Yin (d)	⬜

You are one of the four following combinations:
A Lesser Yang and Greater Yin combination is called YangYin.
A Lesser Yang and Greater Yang combination is called YangYang.
A Lesser Yin and Greater Yang combination is called YinYang.
And a Lesser Yin and Greater Yin combination is called YinYin.

Pointer #2: about 30% of people answering the questionnaire misdiagnose themselves.

LESSER YANG (A) AND LESSER YIN (B) QUESTIONNAIRE

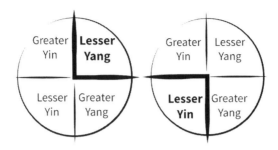

Note: There are 27 questions. The following descriptions pertaining to questions 1 to 18 apply to 100% of the population. About half the population fits one characteristic and the other half fits the opposite. If one description does not apply to you, then the other one does. For each question, you need to check one of the two choices; do not leave them blank.

Oftentimes, both answers to each question may be correct, depending on specific situations, but determine which one describes you the <u>more</u> accurately. The following descriptions are conditions <u>based on your healthy state</u> in the absence of any disease or ailment.

☐ 1a. I find myself almost never skipping meals. If I skip a meal, I get easily agitated and irritated.

☐ b. I often find myself forgetting to eat meals. I skip meals regularly and do not feel strong hunger pangs on an empty stomach.

☐ 2a. I cannot eat slowly. In a group of 10 people, I am one of the first three to finish a meal.

☐ b. I eat slowly. In a group of 10 people, I am one of the last three to finish a meal.

☐ 3a. I am not picky with foods. I tend to try new dishes and flavors.

☐ b. I am finicky with foods. There are many food items or dishes I avoid or refuse to try.

☐ 4a. I like mint flavored gum or candy more than cinnamon.

☐ b. I like cinnamon flavored gum or candy more than mint.

☐ 5a. Generally, I find myself rushing to accomplish tasks at the last moment, instead of in step-by-step increments.

- ☐ b. Generally, I do my tasks in step-by-step increments.
- ☐ 6a. It is a challenge to keep a regular diary.
- ☐ b. I do keep or can keep a regular diary.
- ☐ 7a. I prefer to live without a daily schedule on my phone or organizer.
- ☐ b. I cannot imagine living a smooth life without a daily schedule on my phone or organizer.
- ☐ 8a. It is cumbersome to keep track of detailed information, and I am not detail-oriented.
- ☐ b. I am good at paying attention to minute details; I do not mind it being a requirement of my career.
- ☐ 9a. My room is often disorganized but I can easily find what I need.
- ☐ b. My room is usually organized and I cannot think clearly if it is messy.
- ☐ 10a. I am usually the first person to try something new, rather than relying on someone else to be a guinea pig.
- ☐ b. I would rather have somebody else try something new before I do. I am usually not the first to try.
- ☐ 11a. I have ADHD (Attention Deficit Hyperactive Disorder) or a mild form of it.
- ☐ b. I have obsessive-compulsive disorder or a mild form of it.
- ☐ 12a .When I was a baby, I generally slept through the night.
- ☐ b. When I was a baby, I woke up often during the night.
- ☐ 13a. I can sleep anywhere and sleep deeply.
- ☐ b. I am finicky about where I sleep and am a light sleeper.
- ☐ 14a. When I am extremely tired, I fall asleep very easily.
- ☐ b. When I am extremely tired, I find it difficult to fall asleep.
- ☐ 15a. Caffeine generally does not affect my sleep.
- ☐ b. Caffeine will cause insomnia if I drink it after 3:00 pm.
- ☐ 16a. Even in cold weather, I cannot sleep with a blanket over my face; I feel confined.
- ☐ b. In cold weather, I often like to sleep with a blanket over my face.
- ☐ 17a. My hands and feet are usually warm. When they get cold, they quickly warm back up.
- ☐ b. My hands and feet get cold easily and tend to stay cold.
- ☐ 18a. Drinking ice water does not cause cramps or bloating. I can drink it all day.

- ☐ b. Drinking ice water causes cramping or bloating. It occurs immediately or after a few days of consistently drinking it.
- ☐ 19a. I had a soy allergy as an infant or as an adult which might have ranged from skin itching or to anaphylactic shock.
- ☐ b. Intentionally left blank.
- ☐ 20a. Intentionally left blank.
- ☐ b. I am allergic or intolerant to many prescription and over-the-counter medications. Or I need to take less than average dosage to have the same effect.
- ☐ 21a. Intentionally left blank.
- ☐ b. I am often sick with food-poisoning symptoms after eating out at a restaurant. The artificial flavoring such as monosodium glutamate, artificial coloring, and food preservatives such as nitrites cause headaches, indigestion, and fatigue.
- ☐ 22a. I am allergic or have intolerance to corn. Corn starch and syrup cause arthritic pains and fatigue.
- ☐ b. I have gluten intolerance. Wheat products make me bloated or cause symptoms of irritable bowel syndrome.
- ☐ 23a. Intentionally left blank.
- ☐ b. I've always had thick hair. I have many follicles on my scalp that contain two or three hair roots. My hair density is in the top 20 percentile of the population.
- ☐ 24a. Intentionally left blank.
- ☐ b. I have a history of being anemic (mild to severe) or am prone to anemia.
- ☐ 25a. Intentionally left blank.
- ☐ b. I am or was diagnosed with gastroparesis, which is the slow emptying of food from the stomach into the small intestine.
- ☐ 26a. Intentionally left blank.
- ☐ b. I am or was diagnosed with Raynaud's phenomenon, a condition of extreme coldness and discoloration of the fingers and toes due to lack of proper blood circulation.
- ☐ 27a. Intentionally left blank.
- ☐ b. I have allergic contact dermatitis to latex and/or nickel. My skin breaks out with itching, rash, and redness.

Pointer #3: Having had celiac disease (gluten intolerance), gastroparesis, and/or Raynaud's phenomenon in severe form increases the likelihood of being a Lesser Yin by 95%. A confirmed medical diagnosis of corn allergy likewise makes the likelihood of being a Lesser Yang by the same percentage.

Pointer #4: Severe, tortuous varicose veins in the legs indicate a 90% likelihood of being a YinYin (Lesser Yin and Greater Yin combination). Those who are highly sensitive to trace amounts of artificial food additives and chemicals, manifesting as severe headaches, fatigue, and irritable bowel syndrome, are also likely a YinYin by the same percentage.

Pointer #5: Having severe adverse reaction to most prescription medications indicates the body type as YinYin (Lesser Yin and Greater Yin combination) by 90%. For this reason, YinYins tend to seek complementary and alternative medicine practitioners known for their gentler approach.

Pointer #6: Having severe contact dermatitis or anaphylaxis to latex and/or nickel makes a likelihood of being a Lesser Yin by 80% to 90%.

GREATER YANG (C) AND GREATER YIN (D) QUESTIONNAIRE

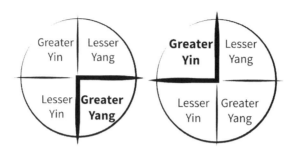

Note: There are 22 questions. The following descriptions from questions 1 to 21 apply to 100% of the population. About half the population fits one characteristic and the other half fits the opposite. For each question, you need to choose one of the two descriptions; do not leave any blank.

Oftentimes, both answers to each question may be correct, depending on specific situations, but determine which one describes you the <u>more</u> accurately. The following descriptions are conditions <u>based on your healthy state</u>.

- ❐ 1c. I find steaks to be heavy and take a long time to digest. My bowels are often affected. I do not like the sensation from eating a high protein diet, which makes me feel heavy, tired, and bloated.
- ❐ d. I do not find steaks to be heavy. I digest them quickly and my bowels do not change. I benefit from a high protein diet, which results in weight loss, and an increase in energy, focus, and clarity.
- ❐ 2c. I find greasy or fried foods to be heavy and take a long time to digest. My bowels are often easily affected.
- ❐ d. I do not find greasy or fried foods to be heavy. I digest them quickly and my bowels do not change.
- ❐ 3c. I get motion sickness easily, such as on boats or airplanes. I cannot read a book as a passenger in a car for more than five minutes.
- ❐ d. I do not get motion sickness easily, such as on boats or airplanes. I can read a book as a passenger in a car for more than 15 minutes.

- 4c. I am lactose intolerant or allergic to milk products. I experience increased nasal discharge, bloating, and or a change in bowel function after drinking a glass of milk.
- d. I am not allergic to milk products. I do not feel bloated or have a change in bowel movement. I can drink two glasses of milk every day without symptoms.
- 5c. My sense of hearing is keener than my sense of smell.
- d. My sense of smell is keener than my sense of hearing.
- 6c. I feel light headed or dizzy when I have a strong mint taste, such as mint-flavored gum, in my mouth for more than 10 minutes.
- d. I do not feel light headed or dizzy when I have a strong mint taste, such as mint-flavored gum, in my mouth for more than 10 minutes.
- 7c. I do not like perfume or strong odors. They sometimes give me a headache or make me feel dizzy.
- d. I am not bothered by perfume or strong odors.
- 8c. Regardless of the quality, my voice is middle- to high-pitched.
- d. Regardless of the quality, my voice is middle- to low-pitched.
- 9c. I would rather be warm than cold.
- d. I would rather be cold than warm.
- 10c. I have difficulty ignoring a nagging pain and it affects my activities.
- d. When I am distracted, I often forget I have a nagging pain.
- 11c. I feel uncomfortable wearing a turtleneck or a scarf around my neck, even in cooler weather. I use it as a fashion statement only.
- d. I feel comfortable wearing a scarf or turtleneck around my neck in cooler weather. I often wear them as a fashion statement.
- 12c. I get bothered if I wear a hat all day.
- d. Wearing a hat makes me feel comfortable and cozy. I can wear a hat all day long.
- 13c. I do not like to talk or to sing for a long time because my voice tends to get hoarse easily.
- d. I can talk or sing for a long time. My voice does not get hoarse easily and my throat is not affected.
- 14c. I do not like strenuous physical activities. I have to put in extra effort.
- d. I like physical activities that require strength or stamina.
- 15c. My shoes tend to last a long time and stay in pristine shape.

- ❑ d. My shoes tend to break down easily, especially on the sides.
- ❑ 16c. I cannot stay awake all night to finish a project.
- ❑ d. I can stay up all night to finish a project.
- ❑ 17c. I prefer to sit and do not like to stand for a long time.
- ❑ d. I can stand for a long time and do not need to sit.
- ❑ 18c. I am a night person. I tend to stay up late and get up late.
- ❑ d. I am a morning person. I go to bed early and get up early.
- ❑ 19c. I tend to act first and plan as I go along.
- ❑ d. I tend to think things through thoroughly and plan before acting.
- ❑ 20c. I am uneasy at heights and it takes time for me to adjust.
- ❑ d. I have no problem with heights and can work in high places with relative ease.
- ❑ 21c. I am allergic to nuts. I have one or more symptoms of scratchy throat, itchy skin, sneezing, throat swelling, or post-nasal drip if/when I consume them.
- ❑ d. I am allergic to shellfish (shrimp, clams, mussels). I have one or more symptoms of scratchy throat, swelling in the mouth, or itchy skin if/when I consume them.
- ❑ 22c. Intentionally left blank.
- ❑ d. I have/had gallstones.

Pointer #7: If you have a life-threatening allergy to nuts and need to carry an epinephrine pen, then you have a 95% likelihood of being a Greater Yang. If you have a life-threatening allergy to shellfish, then you have a 95% likelihood of being a Greater Yin. But an intolerance of shellfish expressed as cramping or irritable bowel syndrome may indicate a Lesser Yin. Removal of the gall bladder due to gall stones impacting the bile duct makes 80% likelihood of being a Greater Yin. But an atrophy of the gall bladder without the presence of gall stones does not indicate a Greater Yin.

LESSER YANG AND LESSER YIN DESCRIPTIONS

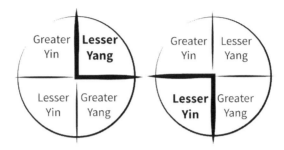

Questions 1-3 and 25:

These questions relate to foods, and the manifestations are multifold. The sensation of hunger is slower to develop in Lesser Yins than in Lesser Yangs. The reason may be that the digestive system of Lesser Yangs can break down food more easily, and their metabolism generally is faster. Usually, once the food empties from the stomach into the small intestine and then to the large intestine, the hunger sensation sets in. Lesser Yangs are more efficient with this digestive process, so naturally the feeling of hunger is quicker and more intense.

This same sensation in Lesser Yins does not register with the brain as quickly. When Lesser Yins are occupied with a project, they may skip meals or forget to eat entirely. Their hunger pangs are not strong enough to remind them to eat. Lesser Yangs, on the other hand, rarely go without eating even if they are busy. The appetite of Lesser Yangs is also relatively unaffected when they are sick or depressed; they can still eat normal amounts of food. When they do not feel well, Lesser Yins may experience decreased appetite or may even vomit. Those who catch the stomach flu recurrently are often Lesser Yins. Gastroparesis, which is a slow motility of the stomach resulting in delayed emptying of foods into the small intestine, is almost always an issue with Lesser Yins.

Lesser Yangs tend to eat faster. They can digest foods well and are not as concerned about indigestion. They may also be physically able to swallow easier with little gag reflex. The ability to swallow is a built-in reflex independent of the size of the person. Participants in eating competitions are often Lesser Yangs. Along with an ability to swallow quickly, their tendencies to appreciate meals with their eyes and quickly register taste are often enough to satisfy them. The result is a developed habit of eating quickly, which they have difficulty breaking. Many Lesser Yangs do not realize that they have overeaten until half an hour later, when the brain recognizes that they are full.

Many Lesser Yins have a strong gag reflex. If a taste is strange, it can easily trigger nausea or vomiting. The accidental slip of the toothbrush into the back of the mouth can also trigger a gag reflex. Many Lesser Yins develop a habit of chewing at least twenty times before swallowing to make sure the foods are broken down enough for their sensitive stomachs to handle. Also, Lesser Yins tend to eat with more emphasis on taste and texture, taking time to savor these qualities, and therefore taking time to swallow.

Although it may be true for anyone, Lesser Yins tend to have a narrow list of preferred foods that they will eat. They are often picky eaters and will eliminate many common foods from their diet. They are put off by strange textures, unusual flavors, and unappetizing appearances. Trying a new dish is not easy for them and they may vomit if forced to eat foods they do not like.

Question 4

Lesser Yins tend to avoid spicy foods because of their sensitive stomachs and tongues, but these items are beneficial to the body. Lesser Yins have "coldness" in their abdomen; warm foods provide relief. Symptoms from mild discomfort to chronic digestive diseases, such as irritable bowel syndrome and acid reflux disease, can be treated with spicy foods. *Helicobacter pylori* is considered the cause of stomach ulcers, but this may be because the person's stomach also creates an environment for the bacteria to thrive. Spices help maintain a favorable digestive environment for Lesser Yins. They get significant relief from common spices, such as cinnamon, black pepper, ginger, and cayenne pepper.

Although spicy foods are not good for Lesser Yangs, they tend to be fond of them because their stomachs are not as sensitive as Lesser Yins, and they like the stimulation. Because of this, they may mistakenly regard spices as beneficial. However, Lesser Yangs have "heat" in their abdomen, so spicy foods actually harm them over time. The easiest way to see if spicy foods are beneficial is to keep cinnamon-flavored candies or other spices in the mouth for a long time. Some Lesser Yangs experience raw, tender sensations on the tip of tongue or a vague discomfort in the head.

Questions 5-11

These questions are related to a cautious nature, which is higher in Lesser Yins than in Lesser Yangs. Not all Lesser Yins are cautious by nature as described in this section, but some are obsessive about it. Lesser Yins are more detail-oriented; they prefer to do tasks step-by-step to ensure that they achieve the desired result. As a precaution, they double-check their work. They start early and do not like to begin projects at the last moment. For this same reason, some consistently arrive early for appointments or meetings.

Some Lesser Yins are deliberately slow, and speeding up to a moderate pace tends to increase unforced errors in their work. They may know answers to examination questions, for example, but still finish slower than others. They are not easily bothered by jobs or tasks that involve repetition. Paying attention to detail is part of their nature. Consequently, jobs that require minimal changes or slow transitions are ideal for them.

Many Lesser Yins turn note-taking into an art form. Their pages are neatly written and well organized. There are rarely cross-outs or erase marks, and their handwriting is legible. Files are habitually kept in order and are marked properly. Self-reflection in diary form is common.

Lesser Yangs are not as cautious as Lesser Yins. They tend to wait until the last minute to begin a task because it is difficult for them to attend to lengthy projects. They would rather not spend additional time working on a project if they do not have to. They see the end first and become impatient if the process is slow. They thrive on jobs or careers that are dynamic and require adaptability. They are often late for appointments or meetings because they tend to underestimate travel time and do not anticipate possible delays.

To Lesser Yangs, taking notes is a hassle that they often view as unnecessary. They are aware that keeping an organizer is a good idea but are not consistent about doing so. Maintaining an updated schedule is not part of their nature. They will abandon a diary or a planner after a short while.

Some Lesser Yangs seem to function comfortably with a messy desk or in a disorganized room. They may appear to thrive in it due to multitasking. Lesser Yangs shift from one interest to another frequently, so many tasks are left unfinished. They move on to other activities, planning to finish the first task later. Although people of any body type might be untidy during their teenage years, some Lesser Yins keep their rooms uncluttered during this time as well.

Extreme cases of these behaviors can be categorized as disorders; these are usually found in Lesser Yins. They suffer more frequently from obsessive compulsive disorder. This is often accompanied by anxiety and depression because they are constantly striving for perfection. At the other extreme, Lesser Yangs tend toward hyperactivity with attention deficit disorder. They are characterized by an inability to stay on task, sit still, be organized, and they have a compulsion to touch things.

Questions 12-15

These questions are related to sleep. Lesser Yins have more sleep problems than Lesser Yangs. Lesser Yins are particular about where they rest and are slow to adjust to new surroundings as they may cause uneasiness. This leads to difficulty falling or staying asleep. A minor worry or excessive fatigue can also prevent restful sleep. In extreme cases, some have insomnia without an apparent reason. This can develop at an early age for Lesser Yins; as babies they tend to be more alert or easier to wake than others. Because they do not sleep deeply, they are also more fretful. As adults, consumption of a caffeinated beverage in the afternoon can cause disrupted sleep in Lesser Yins.

Many Lesser Yangs, especially of the Greater Yin + Lesser Yang combination, often develop a habit of drinking several cups of coffee a day, and can drink a serving of caffeine and still fall asleep within an hour.

Questions 16 and 17

These questions are related to the ability to produce metabolic heat. Lesser Yangs, with their higher metabolism, will burn off calories more readily; this keeps their bodies and extremities warmer. Lesser Yangs tend to get hungry easily and eat frequently. Lesser Yangs rarely have cold hands and feet. Because of their warm bodies, extra exhalation of heat from the mouth and emanation of heat from the face make Lesser Yangs dislike having their faces covered.

Lesser Yins have a slower metabolism and their body temperatures do not run as warm as Lesser Yangs. Because of its inability to produce sufficient heat, the body tries to concentrate it within the torso, so the extremities are the first to show signs of coldness and are slow to warm up. In cold weather, Lesser Yins attempt to conserve heat by wearing socks to bed. Some wear socks every night throughout the winter and even cover their faces and heads with a blanket. An extreme case for a Lesser Yin is Raynaud's phenomenon, where the skin becomes smooth, tight, pale, and is constantly cold to the touch. Cold abdominal skin does not distinguish body type because it can occur in both Lesser Yins and Lesser Yangs.

The ability to retain body heat distinguishes Greater Yins from Greater Yangs. Because Greater Yangs have thinner skin, which releases heat more readily, they get chilled more easily than Greater Yins. Also, the thicker skin in Greater Yins causes dulling of the nerve endings and therefore lessens sensitivity to cold. Individuals with the Greater Yin + Lesser Yang combination have the warmest bodies and feel hot most easily. Conversely, individuals with the Greater Yang + Lesser Yin combination have the coldest bodies and feel chilled most easily.

Questions 18 and 19
These questions are related to the effect of cold-natured foods and drinks on the body and digestive system, as they can quantitatively lower a person's body temperature. Although fats, proteins, and carbohydrates produce heat as a by-product of metabolism, there are other nutrients that contribute to the cooling of the body. Foods are not only for daily function and maintenance; over the long-term, one may see changes in their physiology. Qualitative cold-inducing foods may or may not lower a body temperature, but they will disrupt its normal function, most notably in the digestive system.

Cold-temperature drinks lower body temperature and ability to digest foods in Lesser Yins. Many Lesser Yins find that ice cold drinks cause stomach cramping or bloating. It is infrequent for Lesser Yangs to experience this. For Lesser Yins, warm or hot water with meals aids digestion. If an individual is certain about the negative effect of cold water on his/her digestive system, the person is likely a Lesser Yin. Many Lesser Yangs can consume cold drinks throughout the day and will not be affected at all. A negative response from cold foods or drinks is the only symptom that can be used to indicate a Lesser Yin body type. A positive response or no negative effect is not a definite indicator of a Lesser Yang. Even without the digestive system being affected, Lesser Yin vegetarians experience most notable lowered body temperature.

The quality 'cold' is a functional property in the digestive system of Lesser Yins that makes them prone to indigestion. "Cold-natured" foods can cause digestive problems, such as stomach cramps, indigestion, bowel changes, and bloating. Strong cold-inducing foods are watermelon, cucumber, and gluten found in wheat, rye, and barley. It has long been known in Eastern medicine that wheat has a cooling property whereas rice is warming. This is because of gluten, a protein composite in the wheat and related grains, which causes celiac disease, fatigue, and foggy mental capacity in many Lesser Yins, but not in Lesser Yangs. Many Lesser Yangs do not have trouble eating these foods regularly, while Lesser Yins develop problems with them. Antibiotics are also viewed as cold-natured in Asian medicine. Those who respond slowly to antibiotics or have an allergic reaction are likely Lesser Yins.

Questions 20 and 21

These questions are related to the adverse reactions caused by chemicals in food and pharmaceuticals. Lesser Yins tend to be hypersensitive to many common additives in processed foods such as preservative, flavor enhancer, and coloring. Some examples are aspartame, monosodium glutamate, nitrate, nitrite, paraben, sulfite, and tartrazine. Common symptoms of allergic-intolerant reactions include cough, diarrhea, facial swelling, fatigue, high blood pressure, hives, nausea, shortness of breath, and vomiting.

The adverse reactions from prescription medications are more intense and immediate. Many negative symptoms are identical. Non-steroidal anti-inflammatory drugs, antibiotics, chemotherapy drugs, monoclonal antibodies, anti-seizure drugs and ACE inhibitors cause most allergic drug reactions.

All four body types can have adverse reactions from chemicals in foods and medications. YinYins (Lesser Yin and Greater Yin combination) have the highest negative incidence, followed by YinYangs (Lesser Yin and Greater Yang combination). YangYins (Lesser Yang and Greater Yin combination) are least sensitive and may not notice negative experience as much due to their high tolerance level. Also, YangYins may need higher than average dosage to have the same therapeutic effect.

GREATER YANG AND GREATER YIN DESCRIPTIONS

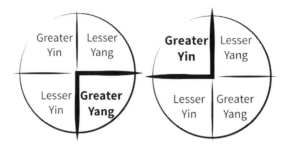

Questions 1 and 2

These questions are related to the body's ability to detoxify itself from heavy foods through liver function and cellular metabolism. Heavy foods are highly concentrated and take longer to break down. Examples of these are fried foods, nuts, meats, dairy, eggs, and beans. Avocados and olive oils are popular alternative oils, but are still heavy. Although bodies can get used to eating these foods over time, there is still an innate difference between the Greater Yang and Greater Yin body types in the amount that can be consumed.

One extreme end of the population can handle a high protein diet well, the Greater Yins. These people tout a low carbohydrate diet consisting mostly of meat, dairy, nuts, and legumes with a positive experience of weight loss, increased energy, mental focus, and mental clarity. If they eat foods consisting primarily of surficial vegetables, especially lettuce and cabbage varieties, then they find that their minds become sluggish, causing difficulty focusing, and even decreased stamina. Many Greater Yins dislike vegetables and leafy greens in particular. Young children react more easily with hypersensitivity to the taste and smell of particular foods. You may remember as a child which foods you found comforting and enjoyable, and also which foods you disliked.

At the opposite end of the spectrum are Greater Yangs, who can handle a low animal protein diet for a long period of time. They feel healthy, their bodies feel light, and they enjoy emotional well-being. They are comfortable with a diet consisting mostly of vegetables and fruits. Consumption of small amount of meats, eggs, and/or dairy satisfy their need for protein. Greater Yangs are not necessarily vegetarians, however.

But they find heavy foods take a longer time to digest and a large amount of them can be quite taxing on the digestive system. They experience abdominal bloating, sluggishness, difficulty focusing, and sleepiness. A meal consisting of a hamburger and fries or a breakfast of sausage, eggs, and bacon can ruin the whole day.

The ability to handle heavy foods is directly related to the body's ability to detoxify, purging harmful chemicals in general. Greater Yins tend to tolerate prescription medications well and experience the desired result with fewer side effects. Their bodies can also handle strong medications and surgical procedures more easily than Greater Yangs because of their high pain tolerance. For these reasons, Greater Yins tend to find Western medical care effective. Many Greater Yangs are very sensitive to over-the-counter and prescription medications. Some react well by taking less than the recommended dosage. Overall, they are more susceptible to drug side effects, even with a low to moderate dose.

However, allergic-intolerant reactions occur most frequently in YinYins (Lesser Yin + Greater Yin combination). For them, it is less about an ability to detoxify, instead pointing to an allergic-intolerant reaction. Rather than defaulting to a higher dosage, small amount of some chemicals can create abdominal bloating, arthritic pain, fatigue, fibromyalgic pain, headache, nausea, and skin rash. Frequent causes are medications and artificial food additives, such as coloring, flavoring, preservatives, and stabilizers. The unexplained discomforts are so strong that they have the most difficulty eating out at restaurants.

Question 3

This question pertains to motion sickness. Common symptoms are dizziness, fatigue, and nausea. They may be caused by repeated speeding up and slowing down in a vehicle. A simple way of testing whether or not you are prone to motion sickness is to consult a map or to read a book while riding as a passenger in a car traveling over a smooth, straight road. Since susceptibility to motion sickness is an inborn trait, it is an indication of a body type. For some Greater Yangs, slight random movements can immediately trigger the uncomfortable symptoms of motion sickness. Even if they train themselves to control these symptoms, the conditioning is quickly lost. Those who remember getting motion sick as a child but seem to have outgrown it are still likely Greater Yangs.

The triggering mechanism in the brain and the inner ear's sensitivity to movements may be less apparent in Greater Yins. These people naturally have greater strength in the abdominal and intercostal muscles, which lessens the symptoms of motion sickness by helping the torso hold steady. Many Greater Yins can read a book in a moving vehicle for more than 15 minutes at a time, while most Greater Yangs have difficulty reading for more than five minutes without experiencing motion sickness.

Those who are comfortable in high-heeled shoes and prefer to wear them all day are also Greater Yins. The reasoning is the same as with motion sickness; they are better able to hold themselves steady and stable.

Question 4

Milk intolerance tends to occur in Greater Yang body types. There are two main ingredients identified in milk that trigger symptoms: the sugar lactose and the protein casein, which are found in cow, goat, sheep, and human milk. Some Greater Yang babies display intolerance to their mother's milk, which manifests as incessant crying, diarrhea, and rashes. The majority of Greater Yangs begin to develop intolerance after the age of five. This tolerance can persist throughout life, but its effect will quickly disappear if dairy is removed from their diet.

Lactose is more commonly the culprit that causes indigestion, gas, bloating, and a change in bowel habits. Lactose free milk is popular with those who are intolerant of this complex sugar. A person who is sensitive to lactose is very likely also intolerant of casein, and vice versa. Greater Yangs do not do well with lactose-free dairy products because casein needs to be removed as well. Removing or minimizing dairy altogether from the diet and finding a replacement source for calcium is necessary for these individuals.

Many Greater Yangs are not aware of the symptoms of intolerance of dairy products and nuts but have chronic hay fever that is triggered by environmental allergens, such as dander, odor, mold, dust, and pollen. The constant presence of dairy or nuts in one's diet makes the body's immune system hypersensitive and makes otherwise mild environmental irritants become major triggering mechanisms.

Many Greater Yins do not develop a deficiency in the enzyme lactase, which helps break down the lactose sugar in milk, even into adulthood. By age five, 90% of the enzyme lactase is no longer present in the digestive tracts of most people, but those who quickly regain it with regular consumption of dairy products are likely the Greater Yin body type.

Question 5

Greater Yins have a stronger sense of smell, both physically and mentally, than the Greater Yangs. They seem to be hard-wired with more olfactory nerves to the brain. The subtlety of taste discrimination lies in the nose picking up odors and working in conjunction with the tongue. Many are comfortable in the field of food connoisseurship. They are cooks and critics of fine foods and drinks.

Greater Yins tend to associate memories and mental processes with the sense of smell. They often use scent related words to describe situations, events, and people. These include words that describe the odors, aromas, scents, and flavors that they experience. For example, the figurative expression "I can smell a pig from a mile away," indicates the way this person places value and importance of this particular sense into the process of thought.

On the other hand, Greater Yangs tend to have a keen sense of hearing and can "hear a pin drop." They have difficulty falling asleep at night if there is even a small noise, such as water dripping, or if their partner snores or tosses and turns.

If both of your senses are keen or dull, try to determine which is relatively stronger than the other.

Questions 6 and 7

These relate to influences by strong or stimulating odors. Many Greater Yangs find mint flavored candies and gums difficult to tolerate after a few minutes. They get dizzy or experience headaches if these are kept in the mouth for too long. The spicy flavor from mint is not the actual cause, but it tends to stimulate the olfactory nerves too strongly and creates an overwhelming sensation in the head. Perfumes and colognes also have the same negatively stimulating effects. A light exposure or a small whiff can cause extremely sensitive Greater Yangs to react with additional symptoms, such as hay fever and difficulty breathing.

Greater Yins can handle odors more easily and many prefer strong aromatic fragrance. They can chew mint gums often and never find them to cause headaches or dizzy sensations. They often wear perfumes or colognes in an amount that is normal to them but others find overpowering.

Question 8

All body types can have a high voice quality and sing well, but the ability to carry a certain pitch range suggests a particular body type. The ability to maintain an extreme pitch at one end or the other makes body type distinguishing easier. Greater Yangs tend to have naturally high-toned voices and therefore can sing in the alto or soprano register. Many Greater Yins have a naturally deep voice with the ability to sing in the baritone or bass range. A person with a voice in the middle range, such as a tenor, can be of either body type.

There are many factors that influence the tone of the voice and can make distinguishing body type somewhat less-than straightforward. Sickness can temporarily change one's voice or can even permanently damage it. Certain kinds of exercise can develop muscles in the neck, thus making voices deeper. Furthermore, a growth spurt can make the voice high pitched and then break. Some people develop a deeper voice depending on social status or for leading a group of people; this is observed frequently in the military.

Question 9

This question is about sensitivity to ambient temperature. Anyone can get accustomed to cold or hot temperatures over time, but there is still an innate preference displayed between the Greater Yangs and Greater Yins. Generally speaking, Greater Yangs get chills easily, whereas Greater Yins can handle—or even prefer—cooler climates. Greater Yins tend to have thicker skin that retains heat better and are able to withstand cold temperatures more easily. For this reason, they can also overheat and have difficulty functioning in the summer months. Those who habitually wear tee shirts and shorts in frigid weather are likely Greater Yins. These people can take room temperature showers or can quickly adjust to the discomfort of wading into cold water.

Many Greater Yangs cannot function well and find it hard to be physically motivated when the environmental temperature is low, especially during the winter. They find themselves wearing more clothing than an average person. Some find it difficult to wear any form of light clothing in the evening or early morning when the temperature is cooler. Before taking a shower, Greater Yangs make sure the water is warm to hot before getting in. Although many Greater Yangs like to swim, they often avoid doing so because of the initial shock of the cold water and their difficulty getting used to the temperature.

Question 10

Thicker skin can sustain more injury and therefore allows for a higher pain threshold. Because Greater Yins generally have thick skin, they can normally handle more pain than Greater Yangs. They seek and enjoy jobs that involve physical labor and exposure to extreme weather. Sports that involve pain are part of their normal active life. For some Greater Yins, it is a stimulant and they do not mind high-risk activities.

Some Greater Yangs have high thresholds, but generally Greater Yins can handle pain better. A person with high touch sensitivity or pain response is likely a Greater Yang due to their thin skin.

Questions 11 and 12

Both questions are similar. Although scarves, turtlenecks, caps, and hats are warming and should be preferred by the Greater Yangs, Greater Yins have more affinity for them. Greater Yangs feel encumbered and find these garments to be bothersome.

Many Greater Yins feel comfortable wearing this kind of clothing. They have a favorite "thinking cap" because they feel they can focus and concentrate better with it on. Some have a habit of wearing accessories on their bodies, such as rings, wristwatches, bands, and necklaces because of their intrinsic value in suggesting a sense of power. Lesser Yins tend to wear them for personal or romantic reasons.

Questions 13-17

These questions refer to a person's strength, stamina, resilience, and ability to recover. Physical athleticism is representative of these qualities. Greater Yins generally are more stoutly built. They have bigger muscles, stronger bones, and better resilience. They tend to be good athletes. Their recovery from injury or surgery is relatively quick.

Being able to stand for a long time without needing to lean, sit, or hold onto an object is a reflection of mid-trunk muscle coordination and whole body strength. The ability to sustain a note when singing or to give a long speech also reflects muscle strength and stability. Many orators and vocalists are Greater Yins. Although some Greater Yangs are also excellent athletes, they generally have to work harder to get to that level.

Physical athleticism also manifests itself in the number of quality sleeping hours one needs. Many Greater Yins sleep only a few hours each night but can function normally and are productive throughout the day. If required, they can stay awake many evenings to work on a project or to meet a deadline.

Greater Yangs may be able to stay awake through one night but will not be able to stay up through two consecutive evenings. They will tire more quickly, so resting the body and getting plenty of recovery time is essential. Greater Yangs can be very productive as long as they are consistent in listening to and abiding by their body's needs.

Question 15

Greater Yins generally have a greater body mass index, bigger bones, and bigger muscles. Because of this, their shoes tend to wear out more quickly. The outer sides of the shoes break down as quickly as the cushioning in the soles. Even with regular usage, some Greater Yins need new shoes every few months.

Some Greater Yangs wear out their shoes quickly because their relatively weaker muscles cause them to drag their feet. Otherwise, however, many Greater Yangs' shoes last for years.

Question 18

Greater Yins generally find it easier to get up in the early mornings and make a habit of doing so. They are the early risers. Their minds work better before the afternoon and they like to get things done before the full break of day. Going to sleep and getting up early helps them to be more productive.

Greater Yangs have difficulty getting up in the mornings and tend to sleep in. It takes them longer to transition from the sleep to wake stage, so their mornings are longer spent getting into gear. They feel more revived after sunset and are more productive until later in the evening. Because they often catch a second wind in the evening, their productivity is maintained until late into the night.

Question 19

This question refers to strategizing with the intention of achieving a better outcome. It is similar to questions 5-11 for Lesser Yangs and Lesser Yins. Organizational skills in Lesser Yins tend to arise more from a fear-based response. The difference is not so much related to the fear of making mistakes as it is a motivating factor, but in the desire to keep track of information. Greater Yins like to strategize and know the step-by-step plan to get to the desired goal before acting. Writing down thoughts and ideas helps them to visualize the task better and have a concrete guide to which they can refer. For this reason, many Greater Yins are avid collectors and keep good records. They enjoy the history, minute details, and trivial facts behind their collections.

Greater Yangs tend to act before thinking through all possibilities and then deal with events as they unfold. They are good at keeping ideas in their heads and are quick to respond to changes. They can easily feel restricted with the notion that their life is run by plans. Both body types dislike chaos and want a sense of order in their lives, though. Greater Yangs and Greater Yins can be efficient at making logical decisions when undertaking large projects and use careful reasoning to execute actions involving minimal risks. The difference between the two is that Greater Yangs are less restrictive on themselves with regards to spontaneous activities, while Greater Yins lean toward making well-thought-out plans.

Question 20
Being comfortable and able to work in high places has two components. One is that the Greater Yin is by nature more physically able to hold steady. The body's ability to keep a stable posture reduces the fear of falling. Greater Yins' sure-footedness results in a lower likelihood of losing balance and falling.

The other component is that Greater Yins generally have less instinctual fear in situations involving risk or danger. Therefore, it is easier for the Greater Yins to rationally overcome their discomfort with heights. Their interests tend to lean toward the arena of conquering, thrill-seeking, and the pursuit to the top. They have less sensitivity to criticism and can better handle stressful situations.

Greater Yangs experience more jitters and prefer avoiding high places. Because of their sensitivity to heights, there are more Greater Yangs who have had bad experiences with these situations. Although the fear of height can be overcome, the training takes longer and the conditioning can quickly be lost without continual exposure to high places. Greater Yangs can also be more easily startled in frightening situations.

Being more cautious and tending to take a safer route is not related to body types. These factors depend on the situation and the individual's assessment of the moment. The social environment and its cues often dictate how we act or what decisions we make.

Question 21

For Greater Yins, eating shellfish can cause minor symptoms, such as a skin rash and itchy throat. A more serious reaction, such as anaphylactic shock—with closure of the air passage and difficulty breathing due to a sudden release of histamines into the blood—strongly indicates this body type. An absence of a negative reaction to shellfish does not necessarily indicate, however, that a person is a Greater Yang because there simply may be no immune response in that particular individual. The presence of an intolerant reaction after consumption of shellfish, such as stomach cramping, but without allergies, skin problems, or anaphylaxis, may indicate a Lesser Yin with or without a Greater Yin aspect.

Those with allergies to peanuts and other nuts are mostly Greater Yangs. Common reactions include itchy throat and itchy skin within an hour of consumption. Anaphylactic shock is even a stronger indicator of a Greater Yang. For many of them, direct and immediate reactions are infrequent, but unexplained skin rashes, chronic sinus congestion, and hay fever are often the result of subtle and delayed negative reactions to nuts that result from continuous exposure.

Skin and blood serum allergy tests on nuts can be useful, but they may not always correctly reflect the true response occurring in the body. Many Greater Yangs have negative test results, but they still have bad experiences with nuts. Chemicals in consumer products, dander, pollen, and dust may be the culprits, but the nuts make the body hypersensitive to these otherwise harmless substances. Even if only one or a few nuts are identified as allergens, that person may still be allergic to all nuts.

Question 22

Having gallstones can be considered an almost exclusive event for Greater Yins. The excess proteins are filtered into the liver, which in turn converts them into bile and dumps them into the gallbladder. This sudden increase will make the proteins aggregate. Increased concentration of bile causes precipitation, forming tiny sand-like crystals that grow over time until they block the passageway.

Gallstones can develop when a Greater Yin loses weight quickly from sickness or from fasting because the sudden loss of body mass is transported directly to the liver. Since Greater Yins tend to be heavier set and consume more greasy foods than Greater Yangs, the liver excretes more bile into the gall bladder. Excessive bile production promotes the growth of stones, causing a blockage of the bile duct. A sudden and severe spasm necessitates the removal of the gall bladder.

An atrophy of the gall bladder, or the presence of sludge within, on the other hand, does not directly indicate a Greater Yin or a Greater Yang body type. Hypo-activity can cause the gall bladder to deteriorate, rendering it functionless. Gall bladder infections also do not necessarily indicate a specific body type because they can occur in everyone.

PSYCHOLOGICAL TYPES: EAST MEETS WEST

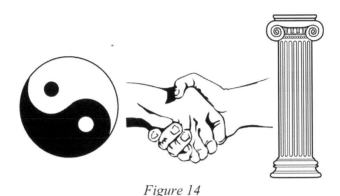

Figure 14

Following the tradition of the four humors introduced by Hippocrates in 4th century BCE and detailed by Galen's four temperaments in 2nd century CE, numerous contributions to their work have been made down the modern age by philosophers and physicians. The 20th century DiSC profiling by William Moulton Marston and Social Styles by David Merrill and Roger Reid have the most direct correlation to the Tetrasoma body types. Myers-Briggs Type Indicator (MBTI), a 16 personality typology that grew out of Carl Jung's interpretation of the four temperaments, also have correlation to the Tetrasoma body types. Although now primarily concerned with personality characteristics and behaviors in psychology, typology is seeing a revival in optimizing health and treating diseases.

Temperament is a person's manner of thinking and behaving, which is an inborn quality and developed at an early age. Temperament is ingrained, expressed as consistent habits across various situations. It is a natural and adaptive behavior demonstrating one's own preferred way of interacting with others. A person is highly predictable based on his or her psychological profile to 80% accuracy. To react differently would require this person to step outside his or her comfort level.

Not all motivations and behaviors reflect a person's temperament. The reason for this variation is multifold: autonomy, environment, family, physiological state, prior events, psychological state, and society are all influencers. People often consciously or unconsciously hide their true intentions, which mask their actual body type. Furthermore, people are constantly evolving to understand themselves through interactions with others in diverse situations. No single characteristic should be focused as a moment that reveals the body type. Rather, the individual should be assessed from a whole-picture perspective that takes into account how they interact in a range of settings.

As you read through the description of each body type below, determine which is important to you, or is closest to your habits as you consider your own motivations and habits. One of the four body type behavioral traits should stand out as your frequent motivator, impulsively propelling you into action.

Form a picture of yourself using all the words rather than a select few. Observe yourself as objectively as possible from a third-person perspective. Make note of which social style you find most frequently expressed in your thoughts and actions. The set of words should be considered together, not as single words, but as groups. To help you identify your type more accurately, form a holistic picture of your behaviors with all the descriptive words, focusing on actions over time rather than recalling specific instances. Do not get hung up on one or two words, but quickly determine which description describes you best overall. Being human, everyone at one time or another will experience all body types in varying degrees. Few words that you strongly agree or disagree with do not necessarily include or exclude you from that body type because the level of characteristics varies from person to person within the same body type. The whole set that stands out most strongly, especially in social settings, will best identify your body type.

Remember that habits are behaviors you find yourself doing often, whereas what is more important may be a value judgment to what you like to be or do. Value judgments may not reflect your body type as accurately because they are often ideas that are contrary your make-up. Your value reaction to some words is unavoidable and can be perceived as good, bad, or soft. Rather than placing value judgments, let your rational mind determine where you tend toward on a daily basis. These words are intended to describe behavioral tendencies. Each style is neither good nor bad, but can be advantageous or disadvantageous, depending on the circumstances. Likewise, all body types have advantages and disadvantages, but none are better than the others.

Ideally, we would like to be all of the characteristics at appropriate times. It would make us versatile, adaptable beings. Actions would be appropriate for every situation. Some people have a better ability to navigate situations with socially acceptable behaviors. For these, it will be more difficult to determine their psychological type. For most others, it is more evident. Although we strive to be a multi-faceted person in all situations, the way our psychological body is hard-wired makes us respond differently from the way others do. Because we do not have all the same fore-knowledge and are not completely prepared, we react the best as we can but still respond according to the self.

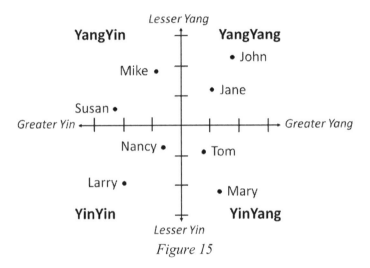

Figure 15

All people fall into any one of the four body type quadrants and will remain in that position throughout their lifetime. It is not possible to shift from quadrant to quadrant. Their body type will remain in the quadrant that they are most innately comfortable in. There is no perfectly balanced person, resulting in everyone being one of four types. The closer one is to the midpoint (x=0, y=0), the less distinct the body type is and therefore more difficult to determine it. The body type imbalance is more skewed as one falls further away from the midpoint, manifesting more of the body type characteristics and making it easier to decide on the diagnosis. It does not necessarily mean that the person is more conducive to sickness and disease. But there will be increased disease when the body type imbalance is not addressed with the body type-specific diet and treatments.

Fill in the bar graphs below with the percentage outcome after you go through each questionnaire.

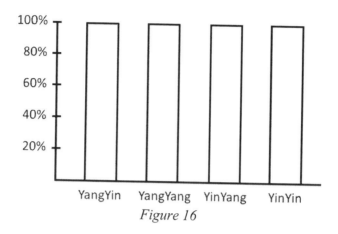

Figure 16

The highest body type score percentage may be your body type. To check if you have gone through all the questions accurately, compare your highest score against its opposite pair. The opposite pairs are YangYin + YinYang and YangYang + YinYin. They are mutually opposite. For example, if you have highest YangYin score, then YinYang score should be least, and vice versa. Also, a highest score as YangYang should have lowest YinYin score, and vice versa. The percentage score for the opposite pair should be the least, and the non-paired body type scores should be between the highest and lowest percentage.

1. YangYin Temperament

(Greater Yin + Lesser Yang. DiSC: Dominance. Social Style: Driver. MBTI: ESTP, ISTP, ENTJ, ESTJ)

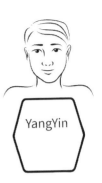

Power, control, dominance, and assertiveness are prevailing characteristics of YangYins. They like to feel a sense of power through controlling the self, others, and situations. They constantly strive to be in power. They take action and get things done. They make quick decisions. They are very quick to use their power and control of situations when dealing with problems and challenges. Since they work best under pressure, their attitude is to readily accept challenges. They are comfortable in juggling many tasks at one time and do them well under deadlines. They are self-confident while not readily displaying emotions or feelings. They come across as able and it is easy for others to rely on them for leadership.

The primary motivation for these individuals is achieving goals through orienting their actions and thoughts toward influence and impact. They take charge, are competitive, and always play to win. They are risk takers and when faced with an obstacle, they try to figure out how to get around it or even go through it, if necessary.

Contrarily, they have fear of being controlled by others and so they take charge instead. Because their fear is failure and they don't like to lose, their actions are centered on winning and getting things done right. They focus on achieving immediate results and ensure bottom line results. They may shy away from details as they do not like to be bogged down with too many steps, which can take away attention from their natural managing talent. They do not like repetition and end up delegating much to others.

The following are typical careers but are not limited to YangYins, who find them challenging and invigorating. Emergency room personnel/high-risk surgery, entrepreneurs, high-impact sports, legal/litigation, operations management, sales – full commission, and sales management. In reality, all four body types, but not as much as the representing body type, can be found in the same profession because there

70

is variation in the particular environment and the job's demand, which can make it suitable.

Those who have opposite behaviors to YangYin body type are described as agreeable, calculating, cautious, cooperative, dependent, docile, gentle, facts-oriented, humble, low-key, mild, meek, modest, peaceful, reserved, timid, uncertain, and undemanding. They cautiously weigh-in and study their options before committing to a decision, shirk from high or risky responsibility, do not like to be in charge, and prefer to be in an affable team environment. They play games for fun, keeping scores only.

YangYin Temperament Questionnaire

Fill in the boxes below with 2 points for strongly agree, 1 point for agree, and 0 points for disagree. Please do not leave any blank as this will skew interpretation of the total score against total scores of other body types.

1. [ ] action-oriented feedback
2. [ ] adventurous
3. [ ] businesslike
4. [ ] candid
5. [ ] challenging
6. [ ] competitive behavior
7. [ ] confident
8. [ ] decisive
9. [ ] delegating
10. [ ] dominating
11. [ ] efficient
12. [ ] empowering self and others
13. [ ] enabling others
14. [ ] fact-oriented
15. [ ] fast-paced
16. [ ] fighting for a cause
17. [ ] forceful
18. [ ] getting things moving along
19. [ ] goal-oriented
20. [ ] greater impact
21. [ ] hard-driving
22. [ ] impatient
23. [ ] impressive
24. [ ] independent
25. [ ] leadership
26. [ ] making decisions
27. [ ] powerful
28. [ ] practical
29. [ ] results-oriented
30. [ ] rough

31.		self-directed
32.		self-reliant
33.		strong-willed
34.		takes charge
35.		takes a definitive stand
36.		takes responsibility for moving ahead and making decisions
37.		task-oriented

High YangYin

In an intense state or in a high-tension situation, this personality type quickly comes across to others who are not YangYins as forceful, impersonal, and independent. YangYins are described by others as: aggressive, argumentative, demanding, determined, domineering, driving, egocentric, egotistical, forceful, pioneering, strong-willed, and unconquerable. They move fast, talk quickly, purposefully make eye-contact, will be the first to extend their hand for a handshake, put their arm around others' shoulders as a gesture of friendship or as a strong assurance, and would rather talk more about tasks to be accomplished than their personal stories.

They are often the weakest listeners of all four types because they feel they do not have time and tend to know the answer. Because they tend to take on too much, they can seem too demanding and insensitive toward others. They are not very diplomatic due to coming on strong and their innate bluntness. They do not like rules and regulations, and are happy looking for loopholes. They frequently challenge the status quo, overlooking risks and cautions.

Following are some of their mantras: "We're going to do things my way," "My way or the highway," "I do not take 'no' for an answer," "Pain is a stimulant to a driving force," "I work through pain," "I want it done right and I want it done now," "Winning isn't everything, it is the only thing."

38.		aggressive
39.		always I-am-correct attitude
40.		ambitious

41.		argumentative
42.		assertive
43.		autocratic
44.		commanding
45.		competitive
46.		decisive
47.		demanding
48.		determined
49.		direct
50.		dismissive
51.		dominating
52.		domineering
53.		driving
54.		egocentric
55.		forceful
56.		harsh
57.		higher status
58.		high risk
59.		impressive
60.		inquisitive
61.		mental fortitude
62.		needs to have the last word
63.		overbearing
64.		overly confident
65.		pioneering
66.		pushy
67.		results-oriented
68.		self-perceived grandeur
69.		speaking harshly
70.		strong-willed
71.		unconquerable
Total Score		

Percentage _____ % = Total Score _____ divided by total possible score 142 multiplied by 100.

2. YangYang Temperament

(Lesser Yang + Greater Yang. DiSC: "I". Social Style: Expressive. MBTI: INFP, ENFP, ENTP, INTP, ISFP)

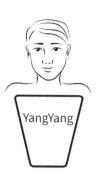

YangYangs are big dreamers, often idealistic. They see the big picture with possibilities of a positive outcome for the benefit of the world. They are great promoters of an idea or a product. People matter because YangYangs want positive impact. They are optimists. Their actions are in conjunction with positive thinking and a sunny disposition. They are all about people. They like to get others involved and be part of a movement. They interact with people well and are highly expressive.

They are generally more willing to make their feelings public. They typically make favorable impressions by participating in a friendly manner. They entertain and generate enthusiasm, motivating people. Their openness to optimism may come across to others as excitement, or a natural gift of persuasion. Their excitement is observable by: rapid speech, exaggerated gestures, rapid eye movements, intense emotion, ability to change subjects quickly, skilled interpersonal interaction, a fast-paced gait, and the desire to share personal stories.

This does not mean YangYangs are extroverts. They can be introverted or extroverted. Extroverts feel recharged when they are interacting in a group rather than being alone. Introverts get their energy when they are alone, rather than being in a social setting where there is a constant interaction with others. The commonality between the introverted and extroverted YangYang is the contagious excitement and idealistic approach to problem-solving.

YangYangs desire to achieve higher standards and to improve personal performance. Because they are not willing to stay with the status quo, their mind is in a good position to make adjustments. The bar in their internal standard of excellence raises once their goals are reached, creating a need to pursue further improvement and refinement.

Their primary motivation is recognition. The achievement motives are enhanced when given praise for jobs done satisfactorily. They are easily stimulated and encouraged by approval. They are most motivated to strive for excellence by applause, praise, and recognition. They want others to be there for them. Their fear is rejection, negative criticism, and disapproval.

Rather than trying to control emotions, a person with this personality will show both positive and negative feelings. They openly communicate their feelings and thought processes, which seem unguarded and revealing.

The following are some of their mantras: "Life is short. Get out and have fun," "Grass is greener on the other side."

The following are typical careers that YangYangs find attractive and invigorating: advertising/marketing, hospitality/tourism, public relations, retail – sales, sales, and training. The values to a group or business are their demonstrative, effervescent, energetic, enthusiastic, impulsive, inspiring, and optimistic behaviors. Some YangYangs are introverted and prefer to be away from the center of attention. They still excel in jobs that are dynamic and do not require a rigid structure to stay focused.

Those who have opposite behavioral style to the YangYang body type are described as calculating, critical, factual, logical, matter-of-fact, pessimistic, reflective, skeptical, and suspicious. They are influenced by data and facts, and not with feelings. They dislike involvement and do not need people to like them. They tend to specialize in one area because they intensely focus on one area of expertise. They concentrate on work content, work alone, are logical, and seek facts. Things matter more than people.

YangYang Temperament Questionnaire

Fill in the boxes below with 2 points for strongly agree, 1 points for somewhat agree, and 0 points for disagree. Please do not leave any blank as this will skew interpretation of the total score against total scores of other body types.

1. [ ] achievement oriented
2. [ ] animated
3. [ ] articulate
4. [ ] attention-seeking
5. [ ] careless
6. [ ] challenge-seeking
7. [ ] cheerful

8.		competitive
9.		convincing
10.		decisive
11.		demonstrative
12.		diverse
13.		dramatic
14.		dynamic
15.		easy-going
16.		effervescent
17.		efficient
18.		emotional
19.		energetic
20.		enthusiastic
21.		excitable
22.		expressive
23.		fast-paced
24.		feedback-seeking
25.		friendly
26.		funny
27.		goal-oriented
28.		gregarious
29.		humorous
30.		idealistic
31.		impatient
32.		impressive
33.		impulsive
34.		inducing
35.		influencing
36.		informal
37.		innovative
38.		inspiring
39.		interactive
40.		less consistent
41.		light, lively
42.		magnetic

43.		medium risk
44.		motivating
45.		multitasking
46.		need to improve
47.		not serious
48.		optimistic
49.		outgoing
50.		people person
51.		performance driven
52.		persuasive
53.		quick to move
54.		decisive
55.		reactive
56.		responsive
57.		seeks short cuts
58.		solo
59.		spontaneous
60.		stimulating
61.		success driven
62.		talkative
63.		trusting
64.		warm

They do not like repetition and do not have patience to do a task repeatedly. When they need to stick with a task, they bring in dynamism to make it interesting and to take the mind off the menial tasks. Rather than being in the now, they tend to project themselves forward toward possibilities. As a result, it can seem impulsive. They immediately look for next thing to do once the goal is reached. Their key desires are maintaining fun, excitement, visibility, recognition, and applause even if this may be an expense of dropping tried and true tasks for the possibility of creating something even more exciting.

They have a problem finishing things. Because they are full of new ideas, they work on the things that are interesting and may leave old projects unfinished. They do not like to repeat things if they have been done once. Rather than mulling over the same information, moving on is preferred. This is why they tend to put off things until at the last minute or before the deadline. They do not like to refine work with repeated editing. They often start things, get bored, and try to get others to finish it or they just drop it. They have difficulty in making formal reports and keeping records. Because they get distracted easily, they can be perceived as lacking follow-through, over-committing, or lacking time-sensitivity. As indicated below, behaviors are more extreme in high-tension situations.

65.		chaotic
66.		cocky
67.		dizzying
68.		egotistical
69.		excitable
70.		flippant
71.		hasty
72.		impatient
73.		impulsive
74.		incomplete
75.		inconsistent
76.		lacking details
77.		late
78.		many unfinished tasks
79.		messy desk, room, car
80.		not gathering enough facts
81.		not serious
82.		over-generalizing
83.		overly colorful
84.		restless
85.		shallow
86.		undisciplined
Total Score		

Percentage _____ % = Total Score _____ divided by total possible score 172 multiplied by 100.

3. YinYang Temperament

(Lesser Yin + Greater Yang. DiSC: "S". Social Style: Amiable. MBTI: ENFJ, INFJ.)

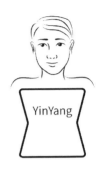

Both YinYang (Lesser Yin + Greater Yang) and YinYins (Lesser Yin + Greater Yin) are oriented toward interpersonal relationships due to their common sharing of Lesser Yin characteristics. These people like to build relationships, networks, and support groups through cooperation and harmony. They are sensitive to the feelings of others and will prioritize these over the task at hand. The main difference between both is that YinYangs place high value on security and YinYins are highly analytical.

A YinYang usually displays feelings openly, but is more interested in being agreeable and cooperative. He or she seeks security and acceptance, therefore maintaining a network of relationships is a primary concern. They are congenial, people-oriented, supportive, and generous with their time. Their activities proceed at a steady pace and are centered on avoiding sudden changes.

YinYang's key desire is harmony. They have strong desire to help others and to be supportive, seeking ways to help others feel good about themselves. They build lasting relationships and show loyalty. They express appreciation to others through words and gifts. Being people oriented, they submit themselves to others through cooperation, patience, persistence, steadfastness, and thoughtfulness. They are great at close, personal, one-on-one relationships and at being reliable team players. They are the glue that keeps a group together. As a consequence, they maintain a network of friends with strong bonds like a family.

Because they are courteous and friendly, they are the best listeners. Their observant behaviors reduce incidence of interruption. They are slower in movement and speech due to wanting others to have their say. They radiate belongingness and a sense of security wherever they go.

Their pace is steady and they perform in a consistent and predictable manner. They make sure tasks are finished before moving on to the next responsibility. They are prone to making mistakes if impatiently spurred or pushed to work on a deadline, although their mental agility is high. Since they are aware that fast physical movement is not their natural inclination, they swerve away from high-pressure tasks or responsibilities. They are resistant to quick change if it threatens relationships.

They have a strong fear of feeling insecure. They like to be in and seek a secure environment. Their problem area is that they often have a hard time saying 'no' because they do not like conflicts and don't want to hurt others' feelings. They may shy away from competitions because of the reality that somebody has to lose. They find themselves going along with a plan even when they really don't want to. They can seem overly tolerant with a depth of patience. They may go along with things while resenting the person even for asking, eventually exploding later when many injustices have been done against them.

The following are some of their mantras: "Don't rock the boat," "Do unto others what you want done to yourself."

They are slow at making big decisions because they do not like change. They like the tried and true, the way it has always been done. They are most comfortable with conventional jobs which are consistent, habitual, organized, prearranged, predictable, prepared, rigid, stable, and systematic. They perform well in a work environment with pattern and develop special skills inherent to the job.

YinYangs tend to seek jobs where it is essential for the society to function, that build long-term relationship and loyalty. The jobs are characterized as being concrete, conventional, cooperative, and having longevity and stability. The typical careers that YinYangs find attractive are, but not limited to: administration/support services, education, finance/economics, human resources, manufacturing, retail – customer service, and teaching/education.

Opposite of YinYangs are those who like change and variety. They like fast-pace circumstances and get bored very easily. They are described as demonstrative, excited, fidgety, frenetic, impatient, impetuous, impulsive, intensive, multi-tasked, pressured, progressive, restless, and zealous. They react to change quickly. They do not like status quo and look for opportunity. They juggle many activities at once, but are not necessarily able to finish them.

YinYang Temperament Questionnaire

Fill in the boxes below with 2 points for strongly agree, 1 points for somewhat agree, and 0 points for disagree. Please do not leave any blank as this will skew interpretation of the total score against total scores of other body types.

1.		accommodating
2.		agreeable
3.		belonging
4.		calm
5.		civil
6.		congenial
7.		consistent
8.		cooperative
9.		deliberate
10.		dependable
11.		diplomatic
12.		does not interrupt
13.		easy-going
14.		emotional
15.		family oriented
16.		fellowship
17.		friendly
18.		friendship
19.		good listener
20.		habitual
21.		desire to keep in touch
22.		low risk
23.		loyal team player
24.		modest
25.		networker
26.		observant
27.		organized
28.		patient
29.		peaceful

30.		people-oriented
31.		pliable
32.		polite
33.		possessive
34.		prearranged
35.		predictable
36.		prepared
37.		relationship driven
38.		relaxed
39.		respectful
40.		rigid
41.		security seeking
42.		sensitive to others' feelings
43.		sentimental
44.		sincere
45.		slow-paced
46.		social clubs
47.		stable
48.		status quo
49.		steady pace
50.		submissive
51.		supportive
52.		systematic
53.		teamwork
54.		thoughtfulness
55.		trusting
56.		understanding
57.		warm
58.		willing

The following words describe extreme behaviors in high-tension situations.

No.	Score	Behavior
59.		acquiesce
60.		avoidance of open disagreement
61.		conforming
62.		dependent
63.		lacking in goal-orientation
64.		lacking initiative for action
65.		overly reliant on relationships
66.		overly subjective
67.		passive
68.		soft-hearted
69.		submissive
70.		too considerate of others
71.		unassertive
72.		not opinionated
73.		unsure
Total Score		

Percentage _____ % = Total Score _____ divided by total possible score 146 multiplied by 100.

4. YinYin Temperament

(Lesser Yin + Greater Yin. DiSC: "C". Social Style: Analytical. MBTI: ISTJ, ISFJ, ESFJ, INTJ)

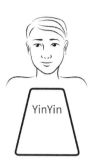

YinYins have natural inclination toward compliance, abiding by rules and policy. They exercise caution and conscientiousness. They tend to gravitate toward analytical behavior without being decisive or forceful. While controlling emotions, they tend to ask questions, gather facts, and study data seriously. Their approach is structured and organized.

The primary motivation for these individuals is quality work. They place priority on getting things right through orderliness and policy. They focus on quality and accuracy through thinking analytically and weighing pros and cons. They strive for competence and self-discipline. They want to know all the details, not only the bottom line for making decisions.

Their key desires are order, accuracy, precision, and perfection. They like to do quality work and do it right the first time. If there is no rule book in place, they will write one. They may enjoy adhering to rules, regulations, and instructions. Organization is what they do best. Rather than opinions, they gear toward encyclopedic, fact-oriented knowledge. Their focus on gathering factual information make them great planners, problem solvers, and organizers. Having considered many facets to a problem, they become great at creating systems. They are recognized as highly inventive and the most intellectual. It is common for them to read manuals and policies from cover to cover.

They exercise diplomacy with people using skill in managing people, handling situations without ill effect. They are quick to think and slow to speak from the desire to avoid conflicts.

They fear being wronged or getting into trouble. There may be a problem with procrastination due to need to do a perfect job. Sometimes they suffer from paralysis by analysis, which is a difficulty in putting into action due to a constant need to gather information. They do not like unpredictable people, disorganized environments, and incomplete or unorganized directions. They are not very outgoing due to lack of spontaneity. High standard of quality often leads to the preference to work alone.

The following are some of their mantras: "Knowledge is power," "The chain is as strong as its weakest link," "Do not leave any stone unturned," "If everybody follows the rules, there will be no conflict," "Everything in its place, and a place for everything," "Get things done right the first time."

The following are typical careers that YinYins find reflecting of their values: accounting/auditor, analyst, computer programming, engineer, editor, quality assurance/safety, research and development, and scientist. Some famous YinYins are Albert Einstein, Leonardo Da Vinci, and Michelangelo.

Those who behave opposite to YinYins challenge the rules and want independence. They will throw a rule book out the window. They are described as acting independently, acting without precedence, arbitrary, assuming authority, careless, defiant, facing up to trouble, fearless, free-spirited, opinionated, rebellious, revolutionary, sarcastic, stubborn, unconcerned with details, undiplomatic, uninhibited, and unsystematic. They like to do things in their own time and in their own way without systematic self-control.

YinYin Temperament Questionnaire

Fill in the boxes below with 2 points for strongly agree, 1 points for somewhat agree, and 0 points for disagree. Please do not leave any blank as this will skew interpretation of the total score against total scores of other body types.

1.		accurate
2.		agreeable
3.		analytical
4.		anticipative
5.		calculating
6.		careful
7.		cautious
8.		collected response
9.		competent
10.		concerned
11.		conscientious
12.		conservative
13.		consistent
14.		contemplative
15.		cool demeanor
16.		cooperative
17.		critical
18.		data-gathering
19.		deliberate
20.		detail-oriented
21.		diligent
22.		diplomatic
23.		double-checking
24.		down-to-earth
25.		exacting
26.		extracting
27.		fact-oriented
28.		focused
29.		follows directions

30.		impersonal
31.		industrious
32.		keeping track
33.		logical
34.		low-key
35.		low risk
36.		mechanical
37.		methodical
38.		meticulous
39.		mild
40.		modest
41.		neat
42.		objective
43.		open-minded
44.		orderly
45.		organized
46.		painstaking
47.		patient
48.		peaceful
49.		perfectionist
50.		persistent
51.		precise
52.		punctual
53.		quality work
54.		quality-conscious
55.		quiet
56.		reserved
57.		rule-abiding
58.		serious
59.		slow-paced
60.		structured
61.		supportive
62.		systematic
63.		tactful
64.		task-orientated

88

65.		technical
66.		thinking it through
67.		thorough
68.		undemanding
69.		wary
70.		willing to listen

In high-tension situations, YinYin traits are exaggerated. The following words describe extreme behaviors across situations.

71.		impersonal approach
72.		indecisive
73.		overly detailed
74.		picky
75.		stiff
76.		stuffy
77.		unresponsive
78.		indecisive
79.		lack of enthusiasm
80.		overly analytical
81.		overly objective
82.		serious
83.		unwilling to take risks
Total Score		

Percentage _____ % = Total Score _____ divided by total possible score 166 multiplied by 100.

RESOURCES

Choi, Seunghoon. *Longevity and Life Preservation in Eastern Medicine.* Seoul: Kyung Hee University Press, 2009.

Merrill, David and Roger Reid. *Personal Styles and Effective Performance.* Pennsylvania: Chilton Book Company, 1981.

New, David and David Cormack. *Why did I do that?: Understanding and Mastering your Motives.* London: Hodder and Stoughton, 1997.

Rolfe, Randy. *The Four Temperaments: A Rediscovery of the Ancient Way of Understanding Health and Character.* New York: Marlowe and Company, 2002.

Rohm, Robert. *Positive Personality Profiles: D-i-S-C-over Personality Insights to Understand Yourself and Others!* Atlanta: Personality Insights, Inc., 2000.

Myers, Isabel Briggs and Peter Myers. *Gifts Differing: Understanding Personality Type.* Palo Alto: Psychologists Press, 1980.

GLOSSARY

Body Type – an inborn nature that is similar or identical to one group but is different from another. It is used synonymously with the word constitution.

Constitution – look up Body Type

Greater Yang – one of four sub-body types and one of two yang types.

Greater Yin - one of four sub-body types and one of two yin types.

Lesser Yang - one of four sub-body types and one of two yang types.

Lesser Yang and Greater Yang - one of four body types consisting of two sub-body types

Lesser Yang and Greater Yin - one of four body types consisting of two sub-body types

Lesser Yin - one of four sub-body types and one of two yin types.

Lesser Yin and Greater Yang - one of four body types consisting of two sub-body types

Lesser Yin and Greater Yin - one of four body types consisting of two sub-body types

Tetrasoma – A four body typology in Eastern medicine that unifies acupuncture, magnet therapy, dietary adjustment, and Western temperaments.

YangYang – short name for Lesser Yang and Greater Yang sub-body type combination.

YangYin - short name for Lesser Yang and Greater Yin sub-body type combination.

YinYang - short name for Lesser Yin and Greater Yang sub-body type combination.

YinYin - short name for Lesser Yin and Greater Yin sub-body type combination

Made in the USA
San Bernardino, CA
07 April 2016